Praise for *Vaccines, Autoimmunity, and the Changing Nature of Childhood Illness*

"Dr. Tom Cowan has created an entertaining, compelling, and readily accessible book explaining the risks involved in today's overaggressive vaccination campaign. I particularly appreciate his emphasis on the risks to autoimmune disease inherent in antibody induction through vaccines. This book is a great addition to the growing body of literature revealing why vaccination is not the best strategy for protection against infectious diseases."

— STEPHANIE SENEFF, senior research scientist,
MIT Computer Science and Artificial Intelligence Laboratory

"I would like to thank Dr. Tom Cowan for writing this book! Humanity seems to have forgotten that human body is part of nature; the further we move away from nature the sicker we become, and it is our children who pay the heaviest price for what modern civilization is doing to our environment and our bodies. This book will make the reader think. I warmly recommend it!"

— NATASHA CAMPBELL-MCBRIDE, MD,
author of *Gut and Psychology Syndrome*

"Tom Cowan's *Vaccines, Autoimmunity, and the Changing Nature of Childhood Illness* is both brilliant and beautifully simple. He shares facts not taught in medical school, that reflect ancient wisdom, common sense, and trust in the intelligence of life itself. Understanding the role of childhood illnesses such as chickenpox and measles is critical to our survival as a species. Tom does an outstanding job of connecting the dots and giving reason to what is often misunderstood!"

— CILLA WHATCOTT, producer of the film
Real Immunity; author of *There is a Choice*

"Dr. Cowan does a great job explaining in clear and common-sense terms that the practice and the rationale of vaccination is deeply flawed, and, astoundingly, is not evidence-based but rather fear-based. The vaccine paradigm is upheld by the consensus, but the consensus in not based on a free and unbiased reading of all the evidence, rather only on a small part of it, while much is ignored. Dr. Cowan contributes greatly to a much-needed correction of this misleading and misled consensus."

— PHILIP INCAO, MD, advisor,
Physicians for Informed Consent

"As a pediatrician for thirty-five years, I have seen the enormous rise in autoimmune diseases like asthma, allergies, eczema, and autism. We no longer need to scratch our heads wondering why, because the reasons are clear. In *Vaccines, Autoimmunity, and the Changing Nature of Childhood Illness,* Dr. Cowan intelligently educates us on the complicated and beautiful workings of our immune system, clearly explains how and why its malfunction is harming us, and elucidates why our precious children are so vulnerable to these diseases. Most importantly, perhaps, Dr. Cowan charts the clear, concise path to healing, offering a better, healthier life for us, our children, and the planet."

— LINDY WOODARD, MD, Pediatric Alternatives

"This book gives parents the intellectual ammunition they need to fight back against the pro-vaccine medical establishment. They clearly need such. I have seen parents driven by fear into vaccinating their children entirely against their parental instincts. By not vaccinating, Cowan shows us how children can be protected from allergy, autoimmunity, attention-deficit/hyperactivity disorder, asthma, and autism. This book is essential reading for all concerned with the health of the next generation."

— DR. SARAH MYHILL, author of
Sustainable Medicine and *Diagnosis and Treatment of
Chronic Fatigue Syndrome and Myalgic Encephalitis*

"This book is a global wake-up call to defend, against those who would destroy it, the awesome wisdom of the human body to wage its own battle against the myriad diseases that seek to overcome our internal defense system. This book will have a profound, beneficial impact on human health around the world in the years and decades to come. It is a courageous and pioneering work worthy of admiration and support."

— NICANOR PERLAS, recipient, Right Livelihood Award

VACCINES,
AUTOIMMUNITY,
and the Changing Nature of
CHILDHOOD
ILLNESS

Also by Thomas Cowan, MD

Human Heart, Cosmic Heart:
A Doctor's Quest to Understand, Treat, and Prevent
Cardiovascular Disease

VACCINES,

AUTOIMMUNITY,

and the Changing Nature of

CHILDHOOD

ILLNESS

THOMAS COWAN, MD

Foreword by Sally Fallon Morell

Chelsea Green Publishing
White River Junction, Vermont | London, UK

Developmental Editor: Brianne Goodspeed
Copy Editor: Deborah Heimann
Proofreader: Nanette Bendyna
Indexer: Ruth Satterlee
Designer: Melissa Jacobson

Printed and bound in Great Britain by Marston Book Services Ltd, Oxfordshire
First printing July, 2018.
10 9 8 7 6 5 4 3 2   19 20 21 22

Our Commitment to Green Publishing

Chelsea Green sees publishing as a tool for cultural change and ecological stewardship. We strive to align our book manufacturing practices with our editorial mission and to reduce the impact of our business enterprise in the environment. We print our books and catalogs on chlorine-free recycled paper, using vegetable-based inks whenever possible. This book may cost slightly more because it was printed on paper that contains recycled fiber, and we hope you'll agree that it's worth it. Chelsea Green is a member of the Green Press Initiative (www.greenpressinitiative.org), a nonprofit coalition of publishers, manufacturers, and authors working to protect the world's endangered forests and conserve natural resources. *Vaccines, Autoimmunity, and the Changing Nature of Childhood Illness* was printed on paper supplied by Thompson-Shore that contains 30% postconsumer recycled fiber.

Library of Congress Cataloging-in-Publication Data
Names: Cowan, Thomas Dale, author.
Title: Vaccines, autoimmunity, and the changing nature of childhood / Thomas Cowan, MD.
Description: White River Junction, Vermont : Chelsea Green Publishing, [2018]
Identifiers: LCCN 2018011990| ISBN 9781603587778 (hardback) | ISBN
   9781603587785 (ebook)
Subjects: LCSH: Vaccination of children. | Vaccination of children—
   Complications—Risk factors. | Vaccines—Health aspects. | Immunization of children. |
   BISAC: MEDICAL / Health Policy. | MEDICAL / Immunology. | MEDICAL / Public
   Health. | MEDICAL / History. | SOCIAL SCIENCE / Disease & Health Issues. |
   HEALTH & FITNESS / Health Care Issues.
Classification: LCC RJ240 .C69 2018 | DDC 614.4/7083—dc23
LC record available at https://lccn.loc.gov/2018011990

Chelsea Green Publishing
85 North Main Street, Suite 120
White River Junction, VT 05001
(802) 295-6300
www.chelseagreen.com

In future, children will be vaccinated with a substance which it will certainly be possible to produce, and this will make them immune, so that they do not develop foolish inclinations connected with spiritual life—"foolish" here, of course, in the eyes of materialists.

—RUDOLF STEINER, *"Fall of the Spirits of Darkness, Lecture 13: The Fallen Spirits Influence in the World," Dornach, Switzerland, October 27, 1917*

CONTENTS

PART III

Treatment and Recovery

FOREWORD

A few years ago, I attended a debate on the subject of raw milk held at the yearly meeting of the International Association for Food Protection, an organization dedicated to pasteurizing, poisoning, zapping, and pressure-treating every morsel of the food we eat, in order to make it completely lifeless and sterile.

The most interesting aspect of the debate was the clear difference in worldview between those for and against raw milk. Those in favor enumerated many of the amazing properties in raw milk—it contains components that protect against pathogens, build a healthy gut wall, support the immune system, and ensure the assimilation of 100 percent of the vitamins and minerals in nature's perfect food.

But those in favor of pasteurization began with a different point of view. "My assumption is not that nature is perfect," said pasteurization proponent Jeff Kornacki, PhD. "My assumption is that nature is wild and can be dangerous." He then referenced the death angel mushroom, which can kill you with one bite—as if to say that raw milk, the magic elixir that has nourished every mammalian baby in the world since the dawn of time—is not just risky, but downright toxic.

Kornacki is typical of scientists and health officials everywhere who believe that nature is dangerous and hostile, and who have constructed their scientific paradigm on the assumption of that danger—danger in the very elements that make our life possible, such as cholesterol and animal fat. Public health officials rail against the dangers of wholesome foods such as red meat and eggs, in addition to raw milk. We are taught that sunlight is the enemy, and our friends, the microorganisms, are out to kill us. According to this worldview, these are mistakes embedded in nature that we must fight against with the newest technologies that scientists can muster.

When health officials assume that nature is imperfect and dangerous, we end up with all kinds of inappropriate procedures—from pasteurization to routine antibiotics to vaccinations. Unfortunately, these are not minor mistakes, but strategies that have led us to the greatest health crisis in the history of the world, and one that has disproportionally impacted our children in tragic ways.

Tom Cowan belongs to a different breed of physician, one who, in the tradition of Dr. Weston Price, makes an alternative assumption: that nature is not hostile, dangerous, and imperfect, but is infused with wisdom. For sure, nature needs a certain amount of thoughtful management to make it compatible with human life, but the showdown confrontation of the physician-cowboy, armed with needles and pharmaceutical drugs, has not made our lives any healthier or happier.

Vaccines, Autoimmunity, and the Changing Nature of Childhood Illness begins with the radical notion that childhood illnesses such as chicken pox and measles play critical roles in the development of our immune systems, conferring lifelong protection against diseases such as cancer and arthritis, and that vaccinations against these childhood illnesses disrupt the immune system in dangerous ways, even introducing chaos into the amazing structural wisdom of the cytoplasm in our cells.

Cowan presents a view of the human body as infused with innate wisdom, and describes a way of supporting and treating both infectious and chronic illness that is born of respect rather than fear. It starts with a nourishing, satisfying diet, provides support for digestion and assimilation, and allows fever to do its important work. Above all, his therapies refuse to incorporate the voodoo science of vaccination and its attendant horrors.

SALLY FALLON MORELL
February 24, 2018

Introduction

When I was growing up in suburban Detroit, my doctor's office didn't have towel racks in the bathroom.

Actually, there *were* towel racks in the bathroom until I began running for them. I would hook one arm through a rack, clasp my hands together, and hold on for dear life.

I was running from Dr. Kuehl, my pediatrician and a friend of my parents, who was trying to give me my shots. My counter-strategy, starting around the age of three, was to run for the bathroom as soon as I entered his office. Since reasoning with me never worked, Dr. Kuehl tried to forcibly pry me loose, but he was left so weak from childhood polio—or, more likely, from a devastating neurotoxicity that was mistaken for polio—that he was no match for an intensely willful kid whose every cell was directed toward the goal of noncompliance.

On two occasions I was sent home vaccine-free. Both times, I agreed to come back another time and cooperate, though I had no intention of doing any such thing. Dr. Kuehl's response was to unscrew the towel racks from the bathroom walls.

This battle went on for years. Every time my mother told me I was going to the doctor's office, it felt like a fight for survival. Sometimes we never even made it out of the driveway.

In some ways, this book is my grown-up version of that small boy's struggle. I haven't, as one might expect, come around to seeing things from the adults' point of view just because I'm now an adult. Or the doctor's point of view just because I'm now a doctor. Far from it. I still empathize with the frightened boy, not the exasperated adults. Dr. Kuehl used to say that he became a pediatrician to spare children the suffering he experienced from polio, but I saw him only as a terrifying adult doing all he could to force me to submit to his dreadful injections. And, although this flies in the face of the deference we're supposed to have for medical authority, I still do see him that way.

I see in my younger self a boy who was right in his struggle. I see a boy who was correct in intuiting that there was something wrong about vaccines—even beyond the momentary pain that probably guided my response when I was three or four, and even though the number of shots I received (or was supposed to receive) was far fewer than the fifty doses that American children now typically receive before the age of six and the sixty-nine doses of sixteen vaccines they receive by the age of eighteen.[1]

And I now realize how correct that young boy was to distrust even those who were ostensibly dedicated to his well-being. After nearly four decades as a doctor, I believe the medical profession is party to one of the most grievous errors a nation has ever perpetuated on its own children. I believe that chronic autoimmune conditions, including autism, are directly linked, though not limited to, the Centers for Disease Control and Prevention's recommended vaccination schedule that most American children follow. And I believe we are in the midst of a massive crisis that is only going to get worse if we don't change course.

As I contemplated writing this book, I had to ask myself why we need yet another book about the dangers of vaccines. Books about vaccines are frequently among Amazon's bestsellers in alternative medicine and pediatrics; many of them, such as *Dissolving Illusions* and *Miller's Review of Critical Vaccine Studies*, are intelligent, thoroughly researched, and convincing, despite what the medical establishment wants you to believe. And there have recently been excellent and informative full-length documentaries, such as *Vaxxed*, that present a chilling and far more nuanced depiction of vaccines than you will ever encounter in the mainstream media. The medical issues are actually easy to demonstrate; there are scores of medical studies in peer-reviewed journals that document how vaccines adversely affect immunologic function. This is so well established that the Department of Health and Human Services has an injury compensation program, specifically for vaccine-related deaths, disabilities, and illnesses, that was established in an attempt to reduce the overwhelming number of lawsuits that vaccine-injured people and their families were filing against vaccine manufacturers and health care providers in the 1980s.

So why yet another book?

The simple answer is that this isn't really a book about the dangers of vaccines, nor a synthesis of the scientific studies, nor an attempt to soften calcified opinions. Yes, I do think vaccines are dangerous and I do think there's abundant evidence to support that stance. There is evidence that our bodies *need* exposure to certain childhood illnesses in order to establish the foundation of lifelong health. For example, in chapter 8, we'll see how a largely benign illness like chicken pox *reduces* the risk of brain cancer, while the vaccine *increases* the risk of shingles. In chapter 10, we'll see how getting measles as a kid reduces the risk of heart disease, arthritis, and allergies. And in chapter 9, we'll see how an innocuous virus that has been with us for millennia, cohabiting benignly in our guts, took the blame for the devastating disease we know as polio—the terror of which helped launch a vaccine manufacturing industry that is projected to be worth more than $61 billion by 2020.[2]

But the larger purpose of this book is an attempt to formulate a new theory on the etiology, or cause, of autoimmune disease, for which western medicine has yet to come up with a satisfying explanation. That is, I'm not only arguing that vaccination is dangerous, though I am arguing that. Or that changing childhood disease patterns—primarily from acute, infectious, self-limiting, and sometimes ultimately beneficial childhood diseases to chronic, autoimmune, and rarely beneficial diseases that often begin in childhood and provoke lifelong suffering—is a consequence of vaccination, either directly or in concert with other environmental toxins, though I am arguing that, too. I'm also attempting to present a framework for how this effect happens. It is a framework in which the gut- and cell-mediated immune reactions such as fever play key roles. And it is a framework that leads inexorably to the impact vaccines have on the structural integrity of our cells.

It's critical for me to point out that I use the terms *autoimmune disease* and *autoimmunity* much more broadly than doctors and other medical professionals typically use them. Some illnesses, like Crohn's disease and colitis, are classic autoimmune diseases with known elevated serum antibody levels. Others, such as asthma, eczema, and allergies, don't have a known elevated antibody level, but there is documented disruption to the balance between the cell-mediated immune system and the humoral immune system (see chapter 3). Further, there is now evidence that the cytokines IL-6 and IL-17 are elevated in certain areas of the brain in children with autism. We also know that these cytokines are elevated as a consequence of aluminum exposure.

In this book, I am describing an autoimmune *process* underlying many illnesses that have their own characteristic imbalance in immune response. Although I often use the term *autoimmune disease*, because I think it's accurate in terms of describing the underlying phenomenon driving so many of these conditions—and that the underlying phenomenon is absolutely essential to understanding, preventing, and treating disease—it can also be helpful to think of these conditions as "immune system imbalance disorders" so as not to confuse them with the more narrow definition of "autoimmune disease" that is used in conventional medicine.

My thinking around the relationship between vaccines, autoimmunity, and childhood, which has spanned decades and includes direct observations of many hundreds of pediatric patients, is based partly on already established fundamental knowledge about how the immune system works, but it is mostly a massive departure from anything you'll ever find in a conventional medical text. For me, it began with remarks made by the Austrian intellectual Rudolf Steiner that have haunted me my entire professional life.

In autumn 1917, Rudolf Steiner gave a series of fourteen lectures in Dornach, Switzerland. In one, he remarked that there will come a time when people will say, "It is pathological for people to even think in terms of spirit and soul. 'Sound' people will speak of nothing but the body. It will be considered a sign of illness for anyone to arrive at the idea of any such thing as a spirit or a soul. People who think like that will be considered to be sick and—you can be quite sure of it—a medicine will be found for this. . . . Taking a 'sound point of view,' people will invent a vaccine to influence the organism as early as possible, preferably as soon as it is born, so that this human body never even gets the idea that there is a soul and a spirit. . . . Materialistic physicians will be asked to drive the souls out of humanity."

In another, he stated that "the spirits of darkness are going to inspire their human hosts, in whom they will be dwelling, to find a vaccine that will drive all inclination towards spirituality out of people's souls when they are still very young, and this will happen in a roundabout way through the living body. Today, bodies are vaccinated against one thing and another; in future, children will be vaccinated with a substance which it will certainly be possible to produce, and this will make them immune, so that they do not develop foolish inclinations connected with spiritual life—'foolish' here, of course, in the eyes of materialists."

Many people find Steiner's work arcane, but the prescience of these remarks has stayed with me since I first encountered them as a medical student, belonging as I do to a profession that has, in fact, reduced itself so radically to such a mechanistic view of the body—and of human experience with sickness and health, life and death—that "sound" people *will* speak of nothing but the body. And there is little tolerance for anything else. Steiner's insights got me thinking about vaccines in the broader context of western medicine and challenged me to try to think *outside* that framework as we witness this dramatic shift from acute childhood illnesses to the chronic, exhausting autoimmune diseases we're seeing in such abundance among children (and adults) today.

American children are now so chronically ill that we must come to new understandings about medicine, health, and disease. We are locked in a cage of symptom suppression like someone trying to stem a flood by holding a finger in the dike. Acute childhood illnesses like measles and chicken pox teach a child's immune system how to respond. Perhaps more importantly, they teach a child how to engage with her body in a powerful and intense way—a process through which a child becomes herself and learns to make her body her own. Preventing or trying to completely control this process will result in a lifelong battle against the self—that is, in autoimmune disease.

If what I'm saying sounds frightening or threatening—or if you jump, incorrectly, to the conclusion that I want to see children die from measles—ask yourself how many children you know with some kind of chronic autoimmune condition. We are *already* dealing with something frightening and threatening: a *massive* epidemic of chronically ill children and a medical establishment that is not only enabling the situation, but profiting from it. If you find yourself wanting to "trust the experts" on this, let me remind you that the Swiss chemist Paul Hermann Müller won the 1948 Nobel Prize in *physiology and medicine* for contributions to the control of yellow fever and malaria... thanks to the use of a marvelous insecticide known as DDT. We cannot survive the current road we are on. We will be too sick, too burdened, too unable to muster enough able-bodied people to care for all the wounded and disabled.

Like Dr. Kuehl, my childhood experiences—including the fear I felt while running for the towel racks—are part of what led me to medicine. And those experiences informed the kind of doctor I became: One who approaches the conventional medical and scientific wisdom with what I believe is appropriate skepticism. One who wonders about the inherent costs of trying to prevent children from experiencing adversity of any kind. One who thinks that when we approach natural systems with brute force, trickery, and a pathological need for control, we usually fail. And one who, after thirty-three years of medical practice, is still asking, "What are we *really* doing to children when we vaccinate them?"

PART I

The Origins of Autoimmunity

CHAPTER ONE

The Changing Nature of
Childhood Illness

W hen I was growing up in the early 1960s, I knew of
one child in our elementary school in suburban
Detroit who had asthma. I remember this distinctly
because he was often teased about his inability to breathe. When
I was in fourth grade, there was another child who died of a brain
tumor. I remember this, too, because of how traumatic it was for
all of her classmates and the school community. Otherwise, I
don't recall any other children who had any sort of chronic illness
or who used prescription medicines. Many of us had horrible
diets, yet chronic disease among children was relatively unknown.
No one had ever heard of autism, let alone had a family member
with autism. Food allergies, to the degree that anyone was aware
of them, were unknown. Peanuts at the ball game were still a
popular treat. Special education classes had not been invented
yet, although there were always the inevitable "slow learners."

I graduated from medical school in 1984 and established a
general practice in upstate New York. A few years later, I moved
with my young family to New Hampshire, where we joined a

vibrant community of other young families interested in Waldorf education, anthroposophy, growing and eating whole foods, and living as naturally as possible. My practice in New Hampshire was one of a number of initiatives that included one of the largest Waldorf schools in North America and one of the oldest Waldorf boarding high schools in the world. We established the first community-supported agriculture initiative in North America, had a strong commitment to the lives and livelihoods of disabled people, and engaged in many other small ventures based on art, biodynamics, and anthroposophy. I was the community doctor there for nearly two decades before relocating to San Francisco in 2003, where I've been practicing ever since.

Because there were many families in that community, many of my patients were young children. Few of their parents wanted them vaccinated, which was fortunate because due to the training I'd had in anthroposophical medicine, I had already come to the conclusion that vaccination and mistreatment of acute illnesses were the primary causes of chronic disease. In fact, the only vaccine I even kept on hand was tetanus, which I've administered maybe twenty times during my entire medical career.

As I developed my practice, I gained considerable experience in the medical care of young children, the age group for which vaccination is most relevant. It afforded me the opportunity to observe children who were in full compliance with the vaccine schedule, those who were in partial compliance with the vaccine schedule, and those who were completely unvaccinated. Because I already had a great deal of skepticism about medical orthodoxy by the time I established my practice—and, indeed, it's why I developed the practice that I did; I could never have tolerated a traditional practice—I can't position myself as an unbiased observer. What I can say, however, is that my observations never caused me to call into question my stance. They only reinforced it.

I rarely saw an unvaccinated child in my practice with a chronic illness of any sort. In general, these children ate healthy diets, played outside a lot, and were in good health. However, among the patients who were partially or fully vaccinated because they'd seen other physicians or pediatricians in the past, I treated many who had one or more chronic health conditions, including asthma, eczema, seizures, and digestive disorders. As time went on, all of these disorders became more common among the partially or fully vaccinated children I saw. I believe this corresponded with the introduction in the late 1980s to the mid-1990s of certain adjuvants and excipients, as well as the introduction of ever more vaccines.

My New Hampshire practice also afforded me the opportunity to treat some of the illnesses for which most children are routinely vaccinated. I have seen hundreds of cases of whooping cough (including in all my three children); hundreds of cases of chicken pox; approximately fifty cases of measles; one case of tetanus; about twenty cases of mumps; a few cases of German measles; no diphtheria; no meningitis; no cases of paralytic polio; and no new onset cases of hepatitis B. Two children in my care were hospitalized as a result of these illnesses: one from complications of chicken pox and one for tetanus. As far as I know, all of the children, including the two who were hospitalized, emerged alive and well, with no long-term complications as a result of their illnesses.

A few decades later, not only is it common for families to have at least one member who's being treated for a chronic illness, but also autism, learning disabilities, asthma, and food allergies have exploded in their frequency and severity. For example, approximately:

> 1 in 2.5 children has an allergy.[1]
> 1 in 6 children has a developmental disability.[2]
> 1 in 9 children has attention-deficit/hyperactivity
>   disorder (ADHD).[3]

1 in 11 children has asthma.[4]
1 in 13 children has severe food allergies.[5]
1 in 36 children has autism.[6]

These numbers represent a national emergency. How is this happening? How, as a society, as parents, as adults and community members, are we *allowing* this to happen? It is a crisis of massive proportions, one that should prompt us all to stop and ask ourselves, "What the hell's going on?" In fact, many of us—as a society, as parents, as adults, as community members, and as individual doctors—*are* asking ourselves that question. But our government and our medical establishment—two bodies that are in the position to do the most about it—continue to act with complacency and fail to acknowledge the severity of this crisis.

Some people claim that this massive increase in cases of chronic childhood illness is the result of better diagnosis. "Better" is an admittedly questionable way to describe current diagnoses; many of them occur when a clinician runs through a checklist on a computer screen, sometimes with minimal interaction or observation of the patient. There are definitely problems with how diagnoses are made, but even overdiagnosis couldn't account for such explosive rates of chronic disease. And while some conditions can be subtle, it is not difficult to identify a child with autism. The behaviors and conditions that lead to an autism diagnosis today were never even reported until 1937 and were virtually nonexistent until the 1990s.

Others claim that these conditions are genetic. It's true that different people can be more or less genetically predisposed to environmentally driven epigenetic damage, but to call this "genetic" is misleading. This kind of genetic predisposition could exist for generations without any noticeable impact on an individual's health until a certain environmental toxin or trigger is introduced. For example, some people are genetically predisposed to clear aluminum toxicity from their bodies less well than others, so these people are more susceptible to damage from an aluminum-containing vaccine. Some will argue that this means a disease is "genetic," but the reality is certainly far more nuanced than that. It would be more accurate to say that a disease is "environmental" with a genetic trigger or predisposition. Framing damage or disease as stemming from an "environmental" cause, however, would require us to do something about it.

The skyrocketing rates of chronic diseases are, in fact, directly linked to the drop in acute infectious diseases, which "train" the immune system. Far from training the immune system in a similar way, vaccination actually thwarts this training with an unhealthy immune response, and does so with the addition of toxins including adjuvants that the body then desperately attempts to clear. We then throw antipyretics—medicines that reduce fever—on top of a by-now-urgent immune response.

Medicine, and in particular modern pediatrics, must take a step back and reevaluate the way it understands and treats children who are sick. A sick child with a fever is not having an emergency. She is going through a valuable learning process, which if continually thwarted will undermine her sacred quest to build a strong body, mind, and immune system for her long journey ahead. Parents and the physicians who care for our children need to throw off the fear-based understanding of acute illnesses that permeates today's medical culture. Today's parents need to be empowered with an understanding of the value of shepherding their children through these types of illnesses. Anytime a fever-reducing medicine, an over-the-counter medicine, or an antibiotic is used when it is not truly needed, a real disservice has been done to that developing child. This change will require not only a new understanding of how our immune system develops but also courage on the part of today's parents to reclaim the human experience of undergoing and overcoming illness. The modern medical promise, often unspoken, is that we are on the brink of a world without disease, pain, or suffering. This promise is misguided and misleading and should be seen as the cruel illusion it is, because it clouds our judgment with magical thinking and renders us incapable of making commonsense decisions. Our children are looking to us—as they should—for wisdom, guidance, and a more sensible way forward into the future.

CHAPTER TWO

Fever and the Nature
of Acute Disease

Give me a medicine to produce a fever,
and I can cure any disease.

—HIPPOCRATES

I n November 1890, a twenty-eight-year-old surgeon named
William Coley amputated the forearm of a young woman
named Bessie Dashiell. A dear friend of John D. Rockefeller
Jr., Dashiell was afflicted with a malignant bone tumor in her
hand. Coley had recently joined the staff of New York City's
Memorial Hospital to work under the tutelage of Dr. James
Ewing, a revered sarcoma specialist, and Memorial was consid-
ered the foremost sarcoma treatment center in the world.
Nevertheless, Dashiell's cancer persisted and spread throughout
her body, killing the young woman in a matter of weeks.[1]

Shaken by Dashiell's death and what seemed like Memorial's
far too frequent failures to treat sarcoma successfully with their
advanced—for the time—surgical techniques, Coley began to

analyze hospital records. He wanted to better understand the rates of success and failure over time. And he wanted to understand the factors. The results, he discovered, were dismal. Very few of Memorial Hospital's sarcoma patients ever actually recovered.

The overwhelming failure was what made the curious case of a German immigrant and dockworker stand out. Records showed that the man was admitted to Memorial Hospital in 1883 with a malignant tumor in his neck. He was later discharged, having neither undergone surgery nor showing any further evidence of a tumor in his neck. Fascinated, Coley sought the man out, found him alive and in good health, and asked about his experience. What Coley learned was that while in the hospital waiting for surgery, the man had contracted a virulent case of erysipelas, a grave and painful strep infection of the skin.[2]

Erysipelas is usually accompanied by intense pain, redness, and high fever. In the pre-antibiotic era, it was not uncommon to see temperatures as high as 105 degrees for weeks at a time in a patient suffering from erysipelas. Nor was it uncommon for patients to die from erysipelas. This patient, however, recovered, and his sarcoma vanished. The surgical procedure was cancelled and the man was discharged.

Cases like this are typically attributed to "spontaneous remission for unknown reasons," but Dr. Coley began to investigate the history of fever and the role of the immune system in treating cancer and other diseases. He discovered in the scientific literature that most so-called spontaneous remissions occurred in patients who had had a concurrent acute febrile illness. He also found a history of physicians using fever therapy in the treatment of their patients. And he learned that European doctors were injecting cancer patients with bacterial toxins to induce fevers. In 1891, Coley began to experiment.

In the beginning, he simply injected patients with *Streptococcus pyogenes*, the strep bacteria that causes erysipelas.[3] Among patients who contracted erysipelas as a result of the exposure, approximately 20 to 40 percent died from the infection. Roughly another 20 to 40 percent experienced no noticeable impact on the sarcoma. And roughly 40 percent experienced remission.[4] These results are intriguing and significant, for two reasons: First, for the first time in modern medical history a nonsurgical therapy resulted in the durable remission of a significant number of patients with an otherwise incurable form of cancer. And, second, no matter how successful the therapy, a 20 to 40 percent mortality rate is too high a price to pay. Coley, emboldened, began looking for a better way.

After several years of experimentation, he was able to isolate the *S. pyogenes* endotoxin—part of the outer membrane of the cell wall in Gram-negative bacteria that elicits a strong immune response, including fever—and mix it with the endotoxin from *Serratia marcescens*.

Each of these endotoxins can provoke significant fevers on its own, but since Coley was using only the part of the bacteria that provokes the immune response, he surmised that there would be a greatly reduced risk of life-threatening infection compared to simply injecting patients with live bacteria. Dr. Coley injected this mixture—known as Coley's Toxins—into patients at increasing doses, depending on their tolerance, provoking fevers of up to 105 degrees on a daily basis for a month. Amazingly, Coley's gamble (with other people's lives) paid off. The death rate plummeted, and the benefits of the fever therapy remained.

Coley treated nearly a thousand patients, mostly with inoperable sarcomas, and his toxins—eventually there were thirteen different formulations—were made available to physicians across Europe and North America from the pharmaceutical firm Parke Davis and Company.[5] A 1945 study calculated a 60 percent cure rate among more than 300 cases of inoperable cancer.[6] This is astonishing and, in fact, far surpasses anything modern oncology has to offer for stage 4 cancer patients.

For decades, Coley's Toxins were used all over the United States and Europe in the treatment of a wide variety of cancers, but never without controversy, in part because Coley could never quite explain how his concoctions worked and in part because results were unpredictable. As early as 1894, Coley's Toxins were criticized severely by the *Journal of the American Medical Association* (*JAMA*), which declared, "There is no longer much question of the entire failure of the toxin injections as a cure for sarcoma and malignant growths."[7] And James Ewing, fanatically obsessed with radiation treatment, forbade Coley to use his treatment at Memorial Hospital.

Coley's Toxins were outright banned in 1962 when the Food and Drug Administration refused to acknowledge them as proven drugs.[8] The postwar years were, of course, also the early heady days of radiation, chemotherapy, and the cusp of the genetic revolution—a time when treating a sick patient with something as simple as the induction of a fever began to seem quaintly medieval compared to blasting a patient with the latest technological firepower. The medical world had discovered aspirin and acetaminophen (Tylenol) to suppress fevers and had begun routine use of antibiotics. The idea of the human being as a self-correcting organism, with the primal event of producing a fever as its main tool, no longer had a place in the armamentarium of the modern doctor.

The irony is that Coley is now considered the father of "immunotherapy," which was reported by the *Atlantic* in 2016 to be one of the most promising "new" cancer therapies in decades.[9] Medical institutions such as University of California, San Francisco (UCSF), and Stanford are increasing their use of "immunological therapies" in their treatment of cancer patients. Touted as a "new," less-toxic approach to cancer treatment, the therapies nevertheless are often administered without an appreciation for the role that fever plays in immune response. (How this will play out is unclear, but if we are going to go down the road of immunological treatment of cancer, we'd be wise to make a serious effort to understand how our immune systems have become so dysfunctional in the first place.) Standard procedure is still to give antipyretic (fever-reducing) medicines at the first sign of a fever and to give antibiotics and antipyretics at the first sign of a bacterial infection—even to cancer patients undergoing various immune therapies.

———————

What does all of this have to do with the changing nature of childhood illness and vaccines?

Broadly, it has to do with how we're looking at health and disease. Until recently, by which I mean prior to the last fifty to eighty years, there were many ways people at different times and in different places understood disease, but they shared some fundamental similarities. Often, someone was going about her life and was confronted by some sort of noxious influence. Maybe it was evil spirits, or cold winds, or disharmony with her ancestors. Maybe it was bad food or water. Whatever it was needed to be "flushed" out of the body.

The "flushing" is what we today call "acute illness." We (modern doctors), however, have forgotten (or never learned) that acute disease—disease that is typically self-limiting and usually accompanied by fever, rash, and pus—is the primary way the body rids itself of unwanted toxins or other substances. For example, if you get a splinter in your finger and do not remove it, your body may make pus to expel it. The pus is the therapy for the splinter, not the disease to be treated. The splinter, technically speaking, is the disease. If you think of the pus as the disease because it is an infection, you might take antibiotics, but the splinter remains. This mistreatment of acute disease is a fundamental mechanism for chronic disease. In order for a disease to become chronic, there needs to be an insult, often a toxic exposure, and then a suppression of the body's attempt to detoxify.

These days, talking about "noxious influences" sounds naive, even childish. We are much more interested in genetics. We furiously attempt to characterize specific mutations occurring in the cells of a specific tumor. We spend billions of dollars a year doing research on DNA sequences in these distorted cells. We have been doing this work for about five decades, and yet there has been only minimal improvement in the prognosis for cancer patients.

For the thirty-plus years that I've worked as a family doctor, whenever I saw a sick child, my first thought was whether I could help the child through the sickness without suppressing her symptoms. For twelve years, I also worked part-time as an emergency room doctor in New York and New Hampshire, and it was a constant source of frustration to me that I had almost no control over how patients who came into the ER were treated, particularly when it came to their symptoms. Children with temperatures over 99.5 degrees were immediately given acetaminophen to "bring their fever down," sometimes even in the waiting room before I got a chance to see them. Once the fever was suppressed, the child would be evaluated to see if he had signs of a bacterial infection. If he did—bronchitis, sinusitis, or an ear infection—antibiotics would be administered to "clear up" the infection. These interventions take place thousands of times per day across America, with little thought to the role of infections, fever, and acute illness in the maturation of the child's immune system.

Understanding the role of acute disease, in general, and fever, in particular, in the prevention and treatment of disease would do more to improve the health of our children than perhaps any other intervention or medical breakthrough. Any medical worldview that ignores the role of fever and acute illness in the development of the immune system—as our medical establishment currently does—will also be fundamentally misguided in treatment protocols—as our dominant medical establishment currently is. This is particularly serious in relation to vaccines, where we are dealing with the developing immune systems of very young children.

CHAPTER THREE

Our Immune System(s)

I currently run a practice in San Francisco, and I've noticed that when my patients come to see me, they often refer to their "immune system," usually to point out that they have been sick a lot lately, which for them means their "immune system" is weak. They often don't have much of an understanding of what the immune system is or does and, to be fair, even what scientists thought they knew about the immune system (but mostly didn't) has been upended over the past decade or so by research on the microbiome and the critical role of bacteria to human health. That said, there are certain fundamentals that haven't changed and that are relevant to a discussion about the cause of autoimmune disease. What follows in this chapter is, admittedly, an extremely simplified introduction to an incredibly complex topic, but one that I hope will suffice in order to present a framework for a new understanding

The first thing I tell my patients about the immune system is that we actually have two systems, which, when working together, create robust good health. The cell-mediated immune system is characterized by the activity of the white blood cells. As organisms evolved, this was our first immune system to develop. As such, it is in some ways simpler and more primitive than our other immune system, the humoral immune system. The function of the cell-mediated immune system is to respond, both chemically and by sending in white blood cells, to areas of the body that have been "invaded" by a foreign substance. The foreign substance could be a microbe, such as a virus, bacteria, or fungi, or it could be a toxin, such as aluminum or mercury.

The chicken pox (varicella) virus, for example, typically infects thousands of cells, mostly in the respiratory tract, the first time a child is exposed to it. The body produces chemical messengers to send white blood cells to the area of infection to eliminate sick and infected cells. The white blood cells may simply engulf and digest the infected cells or they may "spray" the cells with nitric oxide to kill or disable them before digesting them. The white blood cells then excrete this waste, usually via elimination through the skin, hence the pox rash, or through the formation of mucus, which is then sneezed or coughed out of the body.

The crucial point is that with the cell-mediated immune system, the white blood cells' response is the first step in the clearing of an infection or toxin from our tissues. And it is significant that the white-blood-cell reaction involves elimination. The elimination, which may involve a fever, rash, mucus, or a cough, is what we commonly call being sick. In other words, it is the activity of the cell-mediated immune system that gives rise to the symptoms that we associate with being sick. This distinction is vital to understand: It is not the virus, bacteria, or toxin that makes us "sick." These external agents stimulate a response in us, specifically a response of the cell-mediated immune system, and it is the *response* that we call being sick. It is the *elimination* of the inciting event (i.e., an infection) that equals sickness.

A person with a dysfunctional cell-mediated immune system will not get acutely sick. She may die from an overwhelming chicken pox infection with no sign of the infection because her body was unable to mount a defense. And yet thwarting the cell-mediated response is precisely what doctors do when they prescribe medicines or recommend over-the-counter remedies. We *need* a cell-mediated response to clear unwanted invaders from our bodies; that is how we are designed. When patients are unable to mount an effective cell-mediated response or when the cell-mediated response is thwarted with medicines such as prednisone, antibiotics, or antipyretics such as acetaminophen, aspirin, or ibuprofen (Motrin), the outcomes can be devastating.[1]

As organisms became more complex and, in particular, developed hollow digestive systems that were susceptible to invasion by flukes, worms, and other parasites, cell-mediated protection became insufficient. These parasites were often too large for white blood cells to engulf them, and spraying them with large amounts of nitric oxide gas would have been too toxic for the surrounding tissues. So we developed a second immune system. This is the humoral immune system characterized by antibodies that attach themselves to specific proteins, or antigens, on the invader and either destroy them or mark them for destruction by other cells.

With chicken pox, the cell-mediated immune system first clears the invader along with the dead, infected cells from our bodies. This usually takes seven to ten days. Then, through the humoral immune system, antibodies form in response to an antigen unique to the chicken pox virus. This usually takes six to eight weeks. If the child then ever encounters the chicken pox virus again, the antibodies will quickly neutralize the virus before it has a chance to infect any cells. Without infected cells the cell-mediated immune system never needs to get involved, meaning the person won't experience symptoms from chicken pox again.

This twofold response is the basis of our immune system. It is incredibly precise; it is exceedingly rare for a person to contract one of the common childhood viral diseases more than once in his or her life. The antibodies, or at least the blueprint for the rapid production of those specific antibodies, stay with us our entire lives, protecting us from the misery of experiencing the same diseases over and over again.

This twofold response is also the result of millions of years of evolutionary fine-tuning. Interfering with such a precise immune response that has developed over such a long period of time carries with it massive risk of unintended consequence, and should only be undertaken with a great deal of forethought and consideration. Unfortunately, the practice of medicine over the course of the last century is a story of reckless interference with our immune system and, in particular, interference with our cell-mediated immune response.

We have been taught to fear this cell-mediated immune response (i.e., symptoms), or at least to see it as a nuisance. In traditional cultures, the activity of the cell-mediated immunity was often approached with a kind of reverence. Today, we stop it by any means necessary. However, when a child has a fever, cough, mucus, rash, or other symptoms, that tells us that the cell-mediated system is active and could be supported with hot liquids to encourage sweating or herbs to promote expectoration of the mucus and dead cells. Rashes might be encouraged—or, in recalcitrant cases, even provoked—to "come out." Support for the cell-mediated immune system can take many different forms, but the principle is the same: Native Americans' use of sweat lodges; rubbing nettles or Spanish fly on painful joints; venom therapy for arthritis; panchakarma in Ayurvedic medicine; and the ointments and liniments of Chinese medicine. Homeopathy developed as a framework that used small doses of medicine to help the body's cell-mediated immune system clear out the debris, toxins, and killed microbes from our tissues. Traditionally, if a patient was suffering from a chronic disease, curing it involved activating the cell-mediated immune system to "detoxify" the body.

Detoxification is nothing more than a description of the channels the cell-mediated immune system uses to clear debris. As fever treats cancer, the cell-mediated immune system (and its attendant symptoms) is our inner healing channel. And there is a precise process through which this detoxification comes about. All of this changed with the ascendance of modern pediatrics and the introduction of vaccines.

Modern pediatrics is essentially an assault on the cell-mediated immune system. Nothing illustrates this better than the administration of vaccines. Rather than allowing a child to contract chicken pox, we inject him with an antigenic piece of the virus hoping it will stimulate an antibody response without the cell-mediated response. Actually, the catch is that the antigen on its own produces no appreciable antibody reaction, so vaccine researchers have to link it to an adjuvant. This adjuvant can't be a harmless substance like saline because the combination won't produce an antibody response either. The adjuvant has to be an irritant, better known as a toxin. This is the blueprint for all modern vaccines: Isolate an antigenic piece of a virus, combine it with a toxin, and hope for a lifelong antibody response.

As a public health strategy, this leaves a lot of unanswered questions. The first is: If you inject a child with a toxin to provoke an antibody response and at the same time suppress the cell-mediated response with acetaminophen, how will the body clear the toxin? A number of studies have shown that giving acetaminophen, aspirin, or other nonsteroidal anti-inflammatory drugs at the time of the vaccine increases the risk of negative outcomes (and this is also true when they are given to a sick child rather than allowing the illness to run its course).[2] It's the same explanation in both cases: The cell-mediated reactivity is our *only* way to clear these toxins from our tissues. If we thwart the process, the impact of the toxic exposure is far worse.

And is the vaccine-induced immunity identical to the immunity provided by natural exposure to the disease? No, it's not. For starters, vaccine immunity wanes over time, necessitating booster shots. In the mid-1960s, public health officials promised that one measles shot would create immunity for life. We now know this is wrong. You can't bypass the cell-mediated response and at the same time create lifelong immunity.

And, perhaps most importantly, if you're continually stimulating the humoral immune response at the same time as you are suppressing cell-mediated reactions as much as possible, what will the long-term consequences be? Is it possible that stimulating antibody production at the expense of the cell-mediated immunity will result in excessive antibody response? An over-stimulated antibody response is what characterizes autoimmunity. Autoimmunity is a situation in which, for unknown reasons (at least unknown to most doctors), a person's immune system has been activated to produce an excessive amount of antibodies, which react not only to a targeted virus but also to the body's own tissue.

In autoimmune thyroiditis, or Hashimoto's disease, antibodies in the blood see the body's own thyroid gland as foreign tissue, as if it were a virus. The thyroid is tagged and targeted with the same destructive tactics as if it were a worm or a fluke. The symptoms are the result of the inflammatory, destructive response against the tissue and its subsequent dysfunction. Is it so outlandish to ask whether autoimmune disease is a natural consequence of overstimulating the humoral immune response, precisely as we do when we administer a vaccine?

In 2009, researchers at Kobe University in Japan tried to answer this question. They did trials in which they vaccinated different animals according to the current vaccine schedule, and concluded that "autoimmunity appears to be the inevitable consequence of over-stimulating the host's immune system by repeated immunization."[3] This study, while never carried out in such a systematic way in people, complements numerous studies showing that vaccines can cause autoimmune disease and that vaccinated children have higher rates of autoimmune disease than unvaccinated children do.[4]

The connection is straightforward: The deliberate provocation of antibodies without prior cell-mediated activity produces an imbalance in our immune system and a state of excessive antibody production. This excessive antibody production actually *defines* autoimmune disease. So with millions of people suffering from autoimmune disease, at a number unheard of before the introduction of mass vaccination programs, how can this connection be deemed controversial? Vaccines aren't the *only* mechanism for provoking this state of excessive antibodies, but they are certainly one mechanism and, I'd argue, the dominant one.

In this light, changing disease patterns of the last five decades aren't in any way surprising; it's hard to imagine how we could expect anything else.

CHAPTER FOUR

Autoimmunity
and the Gut

In 2017, an English professor of genetic epidemiology named Tim Spector embarked on a three-day sojourn with the Hadza people of northern Tanzania, one of the last remaining hunter-gatherer groups in Africa, as part of a research project developed by his colleague Jeff Leach and reported in an article for CNN.[1] Immediately prior to embarking with the Hadza, he tested his fecal matter for a baseline assessment of his microbiome. While with the Hadza, Spector participated in all their hunting, sleeping, cooking, eating, and recreational activities and ate an astonishing variety of foods: baobab fruit; small Kongorobi berries; underground tubers; the heart, lung, and liver of two hunted porcupines; the larva-filled honeycomb harvested from high up in a baobab tree; and much more. After three days, Spector returned home to England, retested his microbiome, and discovered an astonishing 20 percent increase in its diversity after only three days of following a hunter-gatherer diet and lifestyle. Days later, it reverted to the less diverse—and less healthy—microbiome he hosted prior to embarking with the Hadza.[2]

What's equally remarkable is that while with the Hadza, Spector enjoyed only a small sample of the 600 different species of plants and animals they consume. By comparison, most westerners have an impoverished diet with respect to diversity, despite the abundance with respect to amount. This lack of diversity is significant to autoimmune disease. Autoimmune disease begins in the gut, and treatment depends on the restoration of the gut microbiome and its diversity of species. While few of us will be able to emulate the Hadza in the richness of their alimentary diversity, even comparatively marginal improvements can yield significant benefits to an individual's health.

Thanks to the Human Microbiome Project, we know that the human body contains about two to six pounds of microorganisms and that according to some estimates these microorganisms outnumber our own cells by as much as ten to one.[3] Other estimates put the number lower, but the fact remains that we are home to trillions of microbes, the largest number of which are found in our gut.[4] And while the mapping of the microbiome is complex and not yet finished, we know that diversity is everything. As in agriculture, diversity tends toward a state of health and balance; monoculture tends toward one of sickness and disease.

Starting in our nose and sinus passageways, and extending all the way to the anus, our gastrointestinal (GI) tract is filled with an incredible diversity of bacteria, viruses, fungi, and sometimes larger organisms. The GI tract can be thought of as a long, hollow tube, divided into different sections, each with a different function. The entire tract is covered with a layer of microorganisms, as well as a layer of hairlike protrusions called villi. Microvilli are similar and have some of the same functions, but they can also be found in some other parts of the body, such as white blood cells.

Like our gut flora, intestinal villi (and microvilli) are critical to our health. On the one hand, they enable good absorption of nutrients from the food we eat. Increasing the surface area of the intestinal wall, the villi absorb nutrients and deposit them in the capillaries that lie just below, eventually delivering them into circulation for use as the building blocks of our cells and tissues. The intestinal villi also create tight junctions that result in the selective permeability of the gut wall, preventing proteins, toxins, and other molecules from gaining access to the bloodstream. Like a well-constructed brick wall, the bricks (read: plump, healthy cells) fit perfectly next to one another. Underneath the villi is a layer of collagen and then a muscular wall, which provides structure and stability to the GI tract. The muscular wall is responsible for the contractile movement resulting in peristalsis and the ability to defecate. Without it, the remnants of our food would not move down and out, and our digestive system would grind to a halt.

I often tell my patients to imagine their GI system like a healthy meadow. Healthy subsoil will provide the structure and foundation upon which the upper layers rest. This subsoil is the muscular layer of our GI tract. Then there is the topsoil (the villi), the meadow's nutritive layer; when healthy, this layer provides the nutrients and habitat for the microbial community. In a pasture or garden, a healthy topsoil gives rise to a thick and vibrant grassy layer filled with an incredible diversity of plant life, everything from perennial grasses, wildflowers, and annual grasses to bushes and trees. Moving in and through these grassy plant layers are insects, butterflies, and animals that together create the diverse ecosystem we call a meadow. While meadows may look static, they are, like our gut, teeming with life.

Our gut lining is also home to a diversity of microbial life, forming a carpetlike inner lining of the gut, lying on top of the plump, healthy cells with healthy villi, and supported by the blood vessels and muscular layer of the gut wall. When healthy—whether a meadow or our gut—the various layers work together to create health for the entire ecosystem. This is the basis of resilience, a state of balance and health that accommodates disturbances without compromising the integrity of the whole system.

In our gut, the feedback system of these layers working together enables microbes to synthesize nutrients that are as important to our well-being as the nutrients provided by our food. The gut microbiome has many more functions, such as aiding digestion, providing bulk to the stool, keeping pathogens in check, and perhaps others we have yet to discover.

When intact, these well-functioning layers—in a meadow or in our gut—prevent the absorption of pathogens—a word I'm using to mean anything, including toxins and agricultural chemicals, that causes disease—into the underlying layers. In a meadow, the rich biodiversity and various soil strata help to prevent toxins or agricultural chemicals from reaching the groundwater. Much will be caught and retained by plants and grasses. If this first layer of the meadow is breached, humus in the soil will bind toxins so they can be digested by the worms, fungi, and other organisms in the topsoil. If the topsoil is breached, then the subsoil will act as a physical barrier to prevent the toxins from reaching the groundwater. Of course, toxins will reach the groundwater in plenty of instances; when you overload a system with toxins, it loses its resilient capacity to absorb, integrate, and maintain homeostasis.

When we are healthy, enzymes in the mouth, acid in the stomach, and microbes in the lower gut will often destroy pathogens. If a pathogen escapes these first lines of digestive defense, then the villi will prevent their access to the bloodstream. If the villi are compromised, we have the physical barrier of the smooth muscular layer of the intestinal wall. In health, these systems function together to screen pathogens from the bloodstream. They are, in essence, guardians of our health. On a more metaphysical level, the gut ecology is the preserver of our integrity. We are not supposed to be a teeming collection of unwanted toxins, proteins, antigens, and pathogens floating around in our blood and settling in our tissues any more than groundwater is supposed to be contaminated with toxic agricultural products. When this contamination happens, we set the stage for the onset of autoimmune disease, one of the predominant plagues of modernity.

Back in the late 1970s, I was a Peace Corps volunteer in rural Swaziland, and I remember how disheartening it was to see how eroded the hillsides were. The Swazis valued their cattle above all else. The size and health of a family's herd determined the family's status in Swazi society. Cattle were a sign of wealth, were a guarantee of food, and were used as currency. The country was—at that time—overrun with cattle, the telltale signs of which were the deep hillside erosion from loss of vegetation, the resulting water runoff, and the groundwater contamination from agricultural chemicals sprayed on the corn and sugarcane fields—all ultimately the inevitable consequence of improper and excessive grazing of cattle.

To be clear, holistic planned grazing of cattle or other large herbivores such as that practiced and recommended by Allan Savory is not the cause of soil erosion. Nor were the tremendous herds that graced the Great Plains before the arrival of the Europeans in North America. In fact, over time, appropriate grazing of large herbivores builds up reservoirs of topsoil and can reverse desertification. Overgrazing and improper grazing of herbivores, however, can devastate meadows and grasslands.

First, the grassy plant layer will be decimated. With the loss of ground cover, roots weaken and are unable to hold topsoil in place. As the topsoil washes away, microbial life goes with it. The subsoil becomes exposed and over time is subjected to wind, rain, and other natural elements. As time goes on, large gashes form in the subsoil and the meadow, and the functioning ecosystem dies. This is a catastrophe, not only for the meadow itself but also for the loss of protection against pathogens, especially agricultural chemicals, which will then seep more readily into the groundwater. At this point, without restoration the entire ecosystem collapses. That, to my great sadness, was the situation I witnessed on the ground in Swaziland.

A similar sequence of events happens in our gut. The initial inciting event is a loss of diversity of the microbiome. This can happen in a number of ways. One common way is the failure of a child to go through the birth canal during delivery. Babies are inoculated with the healthy microbes from their mothers' vaginas during delivery and these bacteria essentially function as the seeds that will grow into a healthy, diverse gut microbiome. Babies born via C-section initially host more of the flora found in the operating room than the flora found in their mothers.[5] As a result, many American babies have compromised microbiomes during infancy due to the lack of microbial diversity and the paucity of healthy organisms that should populate their gut. Or, if a baby does pass through the birth canal during delivery, but the mother's vaginal ecology is unhealthy due to poor health, chronic antibiotic use, or yeast infections, the child will start life with poor-quality gut flora and thus develop a poor-quality microbiome.

A typical American child is then subjected to numerous other influences that have a negative impact on the formation of a healthy microbiome. One factor is lack of diversity in the family's diet, especially in the diet of the nursing mother. Another factor is the overuse of antibiotics in medicine and their ubiquitous presence in the food chain. Yet another factor is a lack of foods with healthy bacterial cultures, including lacto-fermented vegetables such as sauerkraut and pickles; and cultured dairy such as yogurt and kefir. These and many other factors, including GMOs and glyphosate (Roundup), create the conditions in which it is the rare modern child who is born with and able to sustain a healthy microbiome. Without a healthy microbiome, like a hillside with no grass, the intestinal villi and microvilli deteriorate, compromising the integrity of our inner ecosystem at the most fundamental (cellular) level.

When a cell is healthy, the cytoplasm is a gel, not liquid, and this is particularly relevant for our intestinal villi and microvilli, as they have such an important role to play in both absorption and interception. This gel state is the result of intracellular proteins structuring the water inside the cell into a healthy, consistently robust structure. (Think of Jello.) Side-by-side cells with healthy intestinal villi and microvilli will prevent toxins and large molecules from gaining direct access to the bloodstream. When the structure and integrity of the cytoplasm are compromised, the cells shrink and lose their connection to one another and gaps start to appear between the cells. Through these gaps, large protein molecules that shouldn't show up in the bloodstream pass through. Once in the blood, the body must neutralize these large proteins by the production of antibodies. These antibodies often cross-react with the body's own tissue, and when they do, autoimmune disease will commence. In other words, the root of autoimmune disease can be found in the "leaking" gut. And the root of the leaking gut is the contraction of the cells as a result of unhealthy gel formation within these cells.

What factors interfere with this healthy gel formation? In fact, there are many, the main one being the loss of or imbalance in the microbiome. There are other factors that directly compromise the cells, including cellular poisons such as mercury, aluminum, formaldehyde, and some agricultural chemicals, including glyphosate. These toxins, including glyphosate, are found in modern vaccines.[6] This process of intoxication results in shrinkage of the cells. Shrunken, distorted cells are the hallmark of celiac disease and other autoimmune diseases. This fact is something that modern medicine is just beginning to appreciate: That is, the etiology of autoimmune disease and allergy can be traced back to distortion of cells and damaged villi and microvilli. And this fact is why diets such as the Gut and

Psychology Syndrome (GAPS) diet and the Specific Carbohydrate Diet (SCD) that focus on gut health and repairing leaky gut are so crucial in the treatment of autoimmune disease, autism, allergies, and other chronic conditions. Both GAPS and the SCD theory identify damage to the microbiome, intestinal villi, and microvilli as the root cause of these conditions.

This relationship between damage to the microbiome and the microvilli and onset of autoimmune disease is well documented in the scientific literature. Dr. Alessio Fasano, a gastroenterologist and researcher at Harvard Medical School, has shown that gluten intake leads to leaky gut syndrome, in which elements such as bacteria, yeast, pathogens, toxins, and partially digested foods get absorbed through the damaged endothelial lining of the gut, activating the immune response.[7] Dr. Sushrut Jangi, also at Harvard Medical School, "found an imbalance of the microbiome in MS [multiple sclerosis] patients such that an immune-suppressing bacteria is up to seven times more abundant in people with MS compared with controls and immune-enhancing bacteria are three times less abundant."[8] Other research implicates damage to the microbiome in a variety of autoimmune conditions.[9]

We are born with an inherent "boundary" in our gut that creates a separation between what is allowed into our bloodstream and what should be kept out. Antigens of all sorts, proteins, bacterial products, heavy metal toxins, and agricultural poisons can breach this gut barrier when the gut lining is inflamed or leaky. This breakdown leads to the production of antibodies that further cellular damage. This process is intrinsic to the process of autoimmune disease.

What does all this have to do with vaccines, which are often administered intramuscularly? The underlying autoimmune phenomenon is the same. And, actually, it has been shown that vaccination does have a direct effect on the microbiome and gut permeability even when given intramuscularly, not orally. The precise mechanism of how this happens is unknown, but I believe that anytime you affect the balance of immune response, you affect the largest and most important organ system of immune response that we have—the gut.

CHAPTER FIVE

What *Is* Autoimmunity?

In conventional medicine, autoimmune diseases—which include such diverse conditions as rheumatoid arthritis, lupus, Hashimoto's thyroiditis, eczema, asthma, Graves' disease, pemphigus, and multiple sclerosis (MS)—are considered idiopathic, meaning that we don't know the causes. That being said, even in conventional circles, there are some aspects of autoimmunity that are considered settled science: There is an "overstimulation" of the immune system such that it produces an excessive amount of antibodies. These antibodies, for reasons unknown, start to cross-react with one's own tissues. This cross-reaction means your humoral (antibody-based) immune system recognizes your own tissues as "foreign" and directs a destructive, inflammatory response at them. It is as if the immune system "thinks" your thyroid (in Hashimoto's or Graves' disease), or myelin sheath (in MS), or lung tissue (in asthma) is an invading microorganism or foreign toxin and brings the force of its destructive powers to bear against this tissue to neutralize and eliminate it. This is an incredible "strategy" against an invading virus or environmental toxin. It is devastating when directed, for example, against the body's own thyroid gland.

As the assault proceeds, symptoms related to inflammation or dysfunction of the targeted tissue manifest. For example, if the disease is rheumatoid arthritis, the targeted tissue is the cartilage in the joints. As the disease progresses, the patient experiences progressive inflammation, heat, redness, swelling, joint pain, and potential disability. If the inflammatory attack is directed against the myelin sheaths, eventually there will be poor nerve impulse transmission and dysfunction of the areas fed by these nerves. If the nerves to the bladder are involved, there will be urinary symptoms. If it's the nerves to the legs, problems with the gait will emerge. In Hashimoto's thyroiditis, the attack is against the thyroid gland, eventually resulting in the gland's inability to produce thyroid hormones. Once this happens, all the classic symptoms of hypothyroidism will emerge.

This is the simple, conventional explanation for an autoimmune disease. The idiopathic part is that there is generally no explanation for why the humoral immune system creates an excessive amount of antibodies, nor why these antibodies cross-react and target our own tissues.

Back when I was in medical school, I noticed strange inconsistencies in the way autoimmune disease is conventionally treated. Consider, for example, two common autoimmune diseases: rheumatoid arthritis and Hashimoto's thyroiditis. Both are antibody-mediated inflammatory attacks on the body's own tissue.

When a patient is diagnosed with Hashimoto's thyroiditis, she's told she has an underfunctioning thyroid and is typically referred to an endocrinologist, a doctor specializing in hormonal diseases. The endocrinologist may prescribe a synthetic hormone—usually levothyroxine, which is sold under the trade name Synthroid—to replace the thyroid hormone and help manage the low-functioning thyroid gland, which will never function normally again. Some patients will experience symptomatic relief, but many will experience little or no difference. An overall feeling of being unwell may persist. I have seen scores of patients in this situation: They feel unwell, they are told it's because of low thyroid hormone levels, they are given a synthetic hormone, and they feel only marginally better. Why? They are being treated as if they have a thyroid disease. Nothing has been done to slow or halt the dysfunctional immune response that is at the root of the underfunctioning thyroid gland.

With rheumatoid arthritis, conventional treatment gets a degree closer to proper treatment by trying to identify the underlying immune response, though its methodologies are still misguided. That is, a patient who is diagnosed with rheumatoid arthritis will generally be referred to a rheumatologist, an autoimmune specialist, rather than an orthopedic doctor who specializes in the treatment of bones and joints. The focus is not primarily on the patient's joints. He is not given joint medicine, joint glue, or joint exercises, except perhaps to relieve the symptoms of joint pain, stiffness, and acute inflammation. He is prescribed medication to prevent his body from making antibodies. Unlike Hashimoto's thyroiditis, in which the focus of treatment is on the targeted organ, in the treatment of rheumatoid arthritis, little attention is paid to the targeted organ, or, in this case, the joints, except perhaps in the short-term acute treatment of symptoms to relieve pain and discomfort.

I've never heard an explanation for this inconsistency. Why is one autoimmune disease—which is solidly recognized as an autoimmune disease—treated like an end-organ disease, while another autoimmune disease is treated as if it's a disease of the immune system?

My guess is that it is a matter of practicality; certain approaches are practical or impractical depending on a given situation. If the immune system is destroying the thyroid, simply wait until the thyroid is more or less destroyed and then take synthetic hormones (or so conventional medicine says) to replace the thyroid's function. If the immune system is destroying the joints, it isn't possible to wait until the joints are destroyed and then replace them. We have to stop the immune system's assault on the joints. What this inconsistency tells me, however, is that conventional medicine hasn't advanced far enough to identify effective treatments that address the underlying immune response—which is at the root of both diseases.

Rheumatoid arthritis may be more squarely treated as an autoimmune disease, but of course the problem with using immune-suppressing medications to stop the assault on the joints—besides the many awful and often serious side effects of these drugs—is that suppressing the immune response doesn't cure the underlying autoimmune disease any more than synthetic hormones cure the underlying autoimmune disease that launched the assault on the thyroid in Hashimoto's thyroiditis in the first place. The immune response is not the cause of the disease. It is the "pus" trying to get the "splinter" out. The rational therapy for any autoimmune disease is to identify the "splinter" and somehow pull it out.

If there is an ongoing immune response, the crucial questions are what antigen(s) is causing the body's excessive antibody response and how did the antigen end up in the bloodstream? Consider celiac disease, in which the sequence of events has been fairly well established: There is damage to the gut (and its microbiome), including to the microvilli, the hairlike cellular structures that protrude from the gut wall to absorb nutrients and prevent leakage. The gut wall becomes inflamed and, over time, muscular and mucosal layers deteriorate, leading to leaky gut. Large gluten molecules are then able to gain access to the bloodstream, where the body tries to neutralize them by making antibodies to identify and tag them for destruction. These antibodies may react with the body's tissue, including the bones, brain, and joints, creating a myriad of both acute and chronic symptoms.

While it's true that antibodies are damaging to our own tissues, they are not the source of the problem. The source of the problem is the leakage of unwelcome proteins into the bloodstream, resulting from damaged microvilli, which are caused by a compromised microbiome. There may be many reasons for a compromised microbiome, including exposure to a poorly tolerated substance—such as gluten.

Treating autoimmune disease, and specifically celiac disease, with pharmaceuticals is an ineffective approach to stopping the tissue destruction and decreasing antibody levels. The medications, which need to be given in huge quantities to have any impact, create a slew of other problems that can include lymphoma, pneumonia, cataracts, and diabetes. They also treat the response, not the cause, of the disease.

Once foods containing problematic ingredients (such as gluten, heated dairy protein, or soy) are eliminated from the diet, the microbiome can heal, the villi can be restored, gluten will stop showing up in the blood, and the body will stop producing antibodies. This strategy reliably breaks the cycle of celiac disease and it should be the model for the treatment of all autoimmune diseases.

There are other explanations for the presence of excessive antibodies in the bloodstream; antibody production is, after all, the goal of vaccination. We now know that stimulating an antibody response without prior cell-mediated activity does not produce the correct type of antibody response. It's not as long-lived and it has the risk of being under- or overactive.

What we are doing when we vaccinate—overstimulating immune response and provoking antibody formation—is what the body is doing in autoimmune disease. We are literally injecting antigens into human beings to stimulate immune response and antibody production and then wondering why so many people have constantly stimulated immune response and antibody production. There is a big difference between this happening naturally in the context of a cell-mediated response and provoking it intentionally while trying to sidestep the cell-mediated response.

It's also worth noting that when the antibodies destroy (or tag for destruction) certain tissues, nuclear material (DNA predominantly) from the cells that make up the affected tissues spills into the bloodstream. This situation also stimulates the body to create antibodies to target the DNA and other nuclear and cellular material, which accentuates the antibody assault on the affected tissue—for example, the thyroid in Hashimoto's thyroiditis. Thus, we see a vicious cycle of antibody-mediated tissue destruction, leading to increased cellular DNA in the bloodstream, leading to increased production of antibodies, leading to more tissue destruction, and so on. Autoimmune diseases are not usually self-healing due to this cycle. Something must be done to break the cycle.

The symptoms a person may experience from autoimmune disease come from two sources. The first is the general imbalance from an altered immune response. This imbalance, in itself, makes people feel tired and generally unwell. Patients with Hashimoto's will often initially present with evidence of increased antibodies—thyroglobulin and thyroid peroxidase—that specifically target the thyroid, but they will have normal thyroid hormone levels. Typical complaints include fatigue, general malaise, menstrual dysfunction, infertility, depression, and insomnia. The symptoms aren't the direct result of thyroid dysfunction; that usually happens later. They're the result of an overactive immune response. It's an interesting moment: We have a glimpse into the symptoms of autoimmune dysfunction—as evidenced from thyroid antibody test results showing a situation that has not yet progressed to full-blown tissue destruction.

An endocrinologist will often tell patients with these initial symptoms to wait until their thyroid starts underfunctioning, at which point they'll prescribe Synthroid. But this moment before full-blown tissue destruction begins is crucial. The patient has an opportunity to change course (see chapters 11 and 12 for my autoimmune diet and protocol) and is much more likely to be successful at this point than when tissue destruction is under way. Once the targeted tissue has been significantly impacted, it will compromise the structure and integrity of cytoplasm, the basis of cellular and tissue health; only when the cells and tissues have the proper structure can they function as they are meant to. When cytoplasm becomes either too liquid or too dry, a disease state is under way. Both ultrasound and magnetic resonance imaging (MRI) can show us when the cells and tissues are compromised in this way and have veered from a state of health. A sampling of patients in my small San Francisco family practice demonstrates the dramatic role cytoplasm plays in my patients' ailments:

The first of a series of four patients was a woman in her sixties with long-standing rheumatoid arthritis (RA) who came in complaining of painful swollen joints, particularly in her wrists and hands. For years, she'd taken an array of toxic pharmaceuticals that are typically prescribed to manage the symptoms of RA, but due to increasing toxicity of the medicines, she was seeking out a different approach and came to me. Leaving aside the autoimmune nature of RA for a moment, let's consider what we can observe in a patient like this. The striking feature of a person with joint trouble is that, in contrast to someone with healthy joints whose bones are separated from each other and cushioned by internal gel-like sacs, the usual gel-like cushions in the joint, such as the cartilage and bursa, are disturbed and leak fluid into the surrounding tissue. The fluid that leaks out is no longer a proper gel but is a less viscous, more watery fluid, which creates the swelling that we see. For reasons I'll discuss later, the joint's ability to maintain water in its proper cellular state is disturbed. That is the hallmark of the disease. It's a state-of-water problem.

The next patient was a young child with a runny nose, congestion in her ears, and a loose cough, the typical signs of an acutely ill child. We could say the child had a "viral" infection, or a bacterial ear infection, but from another point of view the problem was that liquid (in this case, thick liquid we call mucus) kept building up in places it shouldn't have built up. If we were to peer into healthy cells lining the sinus passages, they would be firm, plump cells filled with water in its gel state. In a diseased state, these same sinus passage cells are too warm, the liquid in them "melts," and the fluid extrudes from the cells and carries with it dead bacteria, white blood cells, and other cellular debris. We see this elimination of the "melted" water with stuff dissolved in it as pus or mucus and we say the person has an infection. As in the RA patient, in this child the cell was unable to maintain its cellular water in the proper gel state, the intracellular fluid dissolved, causing the cell to excrete the unhealthy fluid, which in turn created the symptoms we saw as a sinus, ear, or bronchial infection. Again, it was a state-of-water problem.

The next patient was a woman with a lump in her breast, which was diagnosed by MRI and then subsequent biopsy as a carcinoma of the breast. The MRI showed that the lump had an abnormal density, meaning the intracellular water in the cells within the tumor had contracted. The normal intracellular gel state of the water was lost and replaced by a dense, hardened tangle of overly abundant structural proteins. In other words, the central event that was picked up with the MRI was the loss of the normal gel-like structure of fluid within the cells of the breast. Once the gel-like structure of the intracellular water is lost, the cell can no longer maintain its healthy negative charge. A cell without a halo of negative charges is a dysfunctional cell that can't maintain its proper spacing with its neighboring cells. The result is the hard, dense collection of cells that we call a "tumor." One way of looking at this situation is to say the woman had breast cancer. Another way is to say this was a problem related to the state of water in her breast cells.

The final patient was an elderly man with congestive heart failure. In my previous book, Human Heart, Cosmic Heart, *I argue that the heart is not actually a pump and that the reason blood circulates in the body is due to the electrostatic forces emanating from the charged water in the capillaries. If the state of the water in the cells and in the capillaries is healthy and robust, it follows that the flow of blood in the veins back up to the heart will also be strong and robust. If the water starts to lose its charge, the upward flow becomes weak and the fluid in the veins becomes over-whelmed by the force of gravity. The result will be a collection of uncharged water in the lower extremities— what we see in a patient with congestive heart failure. We erroneously blame the heart, whereas the real problem is a problem of "flow." Since the flow is dependent on the charges emanating from water, congestive heart failure can be viewed as yet another problem originating in the inability to maintain water within a healthy, charged state. In other words, like our previous three patients, this man's congestive heart failure was also a state-of-water problem.*

What do I mean by a "state-of-water problem"? For that, we turn to a brief history of modern cell biology.

CHAPTER SIX

Rethinking Cell Biology

In the 1950s, a Danish scientist named Jens Christian Skou solved a mystery of cell biology when he discovered the sodium-potassium pump (Na+/K+), an enzyme embedded within the cell membrane's lipid bilayer. At the time, scientists were perplexed as to why potassium was concentrated inside cells while sodium was excluded from them, when one would expect them to freely diffuse across the semipermeable cell membrane and eventually equilibrate. The search for the mechanism to explain this disequilibrium eventually led to Skou's discovery of the pump responsible for the sodium-potassium concentration gradient.

Considered a crowning scientific achievement, the discovery of the sodium-potassium pump became a foundation upon which other scientific investigation and understanding were built; indeed, much of modern cell biology is dedicated to the investigation of how various pumps and receptors within the cell membrane function. This discovery determined our understanding of how a cell is structured and functions and provided the underpinnings for the research and application of medicines —pharmaceutical and natural—many of which affect the sodium-potassium pump in some way (e.g., digitalis and strophanthus) or stimulate activities in the cell by binding to receptors embedded within the membrane (e.g., opiates and all the hormones).

Perhaps more importantly, the sodium-potassium pump fits into a scientific consensus—one might say a worldview—that has gradually arisen about how we understand the structure and function of cells; indeed, much of modern cell biology is dedicated to the investigation of how various pumps and receptors within the cell membrane function. The study of genetics, with its focus on which chemical messengers turn on or off various genes, is built upon this worldview, which also forms the foundation of the biotech industry and the search for genetic causes and cures for disease. And this worldview also has everything to do with the autoimmune epidemic and the role that vaccines have played in creating it.

Unfortunately, like many things in modern science, the sodium-potassium pump is a myth. Or, more correctly stated, there *is* a sodium-potassium pump, but it doesn't adequately explain the distribution of sodium and potassium. Nor does it adequately explain the negative charge "halo effect" that determines healthy spatial orientation of cells and living systems writ large.

This sodium-potassium gradient is crucial to understanding the working of our cells in health and disease because it is responsible for the charge that surrounds a cell. A cell is like a battery and the sodium-potassium gradient is the charger. This is significant for two reasons: First, only a charged cell is able to do work, just as only a charged battery is able to do work; a cell with no charge— that is, a cell with no sodium-potassium gradient—is a dysfunctional cell. Second, the halo of negative charges surrounding the cell as a result of this sodium-potassium gradient is the most important determinant of a cell's ability to maintain proper spatial orientation relative to other cells. Cells in a proper spatial orientation to each other are healthy, functional cells. Cells that have lost their halo of negative charges are not able to keep their distance from one another and clump together into dysfunctional masses. This dysfunctional arrangement creates disease.

It is my intention to quickly summarize what I think is a flawed understanding and then replace it with a more accurate conceptual framework that connects our cells and our bodies to the natural world in which we exist, a framework in which the cell is a microcosm of the larger world.

———————

Over the past few centuries, scientists around the world have worked out the structure, function, and mechanisms of mammalian cells. Decades of research have shown that the mammalian cell membrane is a lipid bilayer, or two layers of fat with a layer of protein inside. Embedded in this lipid bilayer are various proteins that may act as receptors, as pumps, or in other capacities that help the cell communicate with its environment and carry out its essential functions. For example, there are protein receptors that bind hormones such as estrogen or testosterone. Once a hormone (or an opiate or any of hundreds of other messenger molecules) is bound to a receptor in the membrane, it triggers an action inside the cell.

Once a messenger molecule binds to and activates a receptor protein, a signal is transmitted to the nucleus, which then turns on or off certain sequences of the nuclear DNA we call genes. These genes, through transcription and translation, make different proteins that then create the structures or activities that the particular gene requires. For example, when estrogen binds to the estrogen receptors in the cell membrane, a signal is communicated to the DNA in the nucleus to make the proteins needed to form breast tissue. If the estrogen is removed or the receptors are blocked, this signal will be thwarted and breast formation will halt. Different cell types have various types or amounts of these receptor proteins so that each kind of cell can fulfill its specialized role.

Putting this together, we have a rudimentary description of a cell: We have a lipid bilayer membrane surrounding a "sack of water" (the cell is composed of 70 percent water) in which various components are dissolved, each with a different function. The cell communicates with the rest of the organism through receptors embedded in this lipid membrane. When a messenger activates a specific membrane-bound receptor, it signals activity within the cell. In most cases the activity consists of turning on a segment of the DNA (i.e., a gene or a group of genes) that then gets transcribed and translated into the various proteins that make up the body—some structural, some more functional. The DNA is housed in the nucleus inside the cell and the protein synthesis is primarily the responsibility of ribosomes, suspended in the watery environment in the cytoplasm. The energy to keep this all going is made in the mitochondria with the creation of adenosine triphosphate (ATP).

For a mammalian cell, the high-energy bond contained within the ATP molecule is the currency that keeps a cell running. "Currency" can be thought of as a manifestation of energy that makes something function. If the system is the US economy, the currency that allows it to function is the dollar. ATP is an adenosine molecule bound to three phosphates with a high-energy bond so that when the ATP is "cleaved" into ADP (biphosphates), the energy in the third bond is liberated to do work for the cell. When the second bond is "cleaved," yet more energy is liberated, at which point the one phosphate molecule, AMP (or monophosphate), is shunted back to the mitochondria to be made again into ATP, to be used as more currency. Again, like an economic system, currency is created that can be used to enable a desired activity (such as buying a house), after which one's currency is spent and you have to do something (such as work) to create a new supply of currency to be able to do more activities (such as buy food).

Take the sodium-potassium pump as an example: It is sometimes conceived as a kind of membrane-bound merry-go-round.

There is a binding site on the outside of the pump specific to K+ and one on the inside specific to Na+. Using ATP as its energy source, the pump binds to a K+ outside the cell and an Na+ inside the cell. Once these are bound, the pump spins around and deposits the K+ inside the cell and the Na+ outside the cell. Then the merry-go-round spins again, picks up another K+ molecule outside the cell, an Na+ molecule inside the cell, and spins again—eventually creating the desired K+ levels inside and Na+ levels outside. This differential creates the charge seen on the outside of the cell.

I can't emphasize enough how fundamental this explanation is to our understanding of cell biology and how a cell is structured and functions, and how it forms the underpinnings for the discovery and applications of new medicines and technology. Except, in a fundamental way, it is all wrong. I am indebted to the work of many creative scientists for helping me understand the flaws of the conventional model and steering me toward a more accurate and useful model for an understanding of mammalian cells. (I recommend the work of Gilbert Ling, Mae-Wan Ho, and Gerald Pollack for those who are interested in a more in-depth explanation than I'm able to provide here; see the recommended resources.)

I started to be suspicious of this prevailing model of cell biology more than twenty-five years ago when I was working as an ER physician. In medical school, we learn that cells consist of 70 percent water by weight and that more than 99 percent of the molecules that make up a cell are water molecules. This composition has been confirmed by testing. We also learn that matter can exist in one of three states: solid, liquid, or gas. With water, this is ice, liquid water, or steam. So, in a cell, which of these three states is that 70 percent water by weight actually in? Conventional cell biology tells us that the water is in a liquid state and that the potassium, sodium, nucleus, mitochondria, ribosomes, and proteins are dissolved or suspended in the universal solvent, which is water.

Yet I saw people wheeled into the ER with often terrible wounds, all of which must have involved massive disruption of the cell membranes of whatever tissues were damaged, but I never once saw water spurting out of a wound or a puddle of water on the floor next to a wounded patient. Blood, yes, of course, but why no "pure" intracellular water? Why doesn't this leak out as well? This was one of those instances, we all have them, when the "facts" didn't line up with my observations. I was told, and believed, that we are composed primarily of liquid water, and yet no matter how or where I looked there was no intracellular water to be found within any human being I encountered.

This cognitive dissonance prompted me to start looking deeper into the literature of cell biology. I learned that a lot of what we know about various membrane-bound pumps and proteins has been discovered by scientists using micropipettes—essentially tiny syringes that you can use to poke holes in a cell membrane and even to extract the proteins or the pumps from the membrane itself. To my surprise, I learned that you can poke hundreds of holes in a cell membrane without anything "leaking" out of the cell and, even stranger, without it affecting the function of the cell. How can this be? If the cell membrane creates, as we are told, the basic functional unit of a cell, how is it that we can severely damage this membrane and yet it has no appreciable impact on the cell's function?

In 2001, a biologist named Gilbert Ling published a book called *Life at the Cell and Below-Cell Level* in which he argued that the sodium-potassium pump fails to explain the exclusion of sodium or the concentration of potassium—and therefore the pump can't be responsible for creating the charge across the cell membrane. Ling is a Chinese scientist who earned the prestigious Boxer Indemnity Scholarship, allowing him to study at the University of Chicago, where he earned his PhD in physiology under the advisement of pioneering neurophysiologist Ralph Waldo Gerard. Ling's work is brilliant—and largely disregarded by the scientific establishment. His argument is complex—and I recommend reading *Life at the Cell and Below-Cell Level* for the details—but the core of his argument is simple: The math doesn't add up. While there *is* such a pump in the membrane, it would have to have access to between fifteen and thirty times more energy (in the form of ATP) than is actually available in order to be responsible for the distribution of sodium and potassium. (It would be like having a mortgage payment of $5,000 per month while only earning $1,000 per month. Not only can you not keep up with the mortgage payment, there's no leftover currency to keep the rest of the household running.)

In a series of experiments that spanned decades, Ling also showed that when he punctured cell membranes using micropipettes, it seemed to have no effect on the sodium-potassium gradient or the electrical charge of the cell. Furthermore, he disabled the pump and it had only a negligible effect on the concentration gradient. While there is a pump, and it is embedded in the membrane, its function is more like that of a backup generator, picking up the slack in case the normal mechanism for the Na+/K+ gradient and the charge of the cell becomes disabled.

Ling also demonstrated that the phosphate bonds to adenosine that make up the high-energy phosphate bonds of ATP, in fact, have no more energy than any other bonds between other common molecules. ATP isn't the high-energy currency we thought it was.

This leaves us with a lot of questions. What, then, is the state of water inside the cell? What *does* cause the unequal distribution of sodium and potassium inside and outside the cell? If the cell membrane is actually of limited importance, how do molecules signal the turning on or off of genes? If ATP is not the energy currency of our bodies, then what is the role of ATP? And what then, if not ATP, is responsible for the charge surrounding the cell?

For the answers, we return to my patients in the previous chapter and their "state-of-water" problems: Science tells us that matter exists in one of three states: solid, liquid, or gas. Take copper, for example. Copper can exist as solid copper or copper ores, molten copper, or gaseous copper. Its state at a given time will be determined primarily by temperature, as well as by pressure, and by motion to a lesser extent. So it is with water. Depending mostly on temperature, water exists as ice, water, or steam, each with its own molecular pattern and arrangement.

Defining what state a substance is in no longer involves guesswork. It is easy to examine any substance with a spectrophotometer and come up with a precise assessment of the molecular configuration. Ice has a distinct molecular pattern, water has a different pattern, and steam yet a different pattern. So how is it that water as it exists in a gel-like state has none of these patterns? It doesn't conform to liquid, solid, or gas molecular configurations. As Gerald Pollack pointed out in *The Fourth Phase of Water*, this is because water—and only water—can exist in a fourth state that is as molecularly distinct as the other three states. This fourth, or gel state, is the state of healthy intracellular water in mammalian cells. There is no liquid water in healthy human cells.

The formation of this intracellular gel in mammalian cells is similar to the formation of Jello. In fact, Jello is simply the trademarked name of gelatin, a protein produced from collagen when it is extracted from bones and connective tissues. The ingredients to make gelatin are simple: water and strongly hydrophilic proteins. To make it, you heat the mixture to add energy to the proteins. When these gelatin proteins are mixed with water and energy in the form of heat is added, the proteins unfold, allowing them to form bonds with the water. When this mixture cools, it forms the characteristic gel of fourth-phase water.

Consider human joints. In a state of health, the cartilage, bursae, and internal structures of joints have a form that allows for effective cushioning and prevents the bones from hitting or rubbing against each other. There is a negative charge to the fourth phase of water, so when one negatively charged bursa comes near another negatively charged bursa, they repel each other, ensuring a smooth gliding action with no bone-to-bone contact. Think of how an ice skater glides on ice. The surface of the ice contains a fine gel-like negatively charged layer, which prevents the skate from sticking to the surface. Or if you have ever licked an extremely cold surface that doesn't contain this gel-like negatively charged layer, you know that without the electrostatic and mechanical repulsion, two surfaces will stick, not glide, and your tongue will stick to the extremely cold surface. This is what's happening when someone has bone-on-bone contact, along with its attendant pain and dysfunction.

In other tissues, such as the thyroid, as inflammation starts to affect the organ, we see swollen, watery cells and tissue. Swollen thyroid cells cannot secrete the proper amount of thyroid hormones. Swollen nerve cells, or desiccated nerve cells, are unable to transmit electrical impulses as they should. This change in the structure of the cytoplasm is the pathological cellular hallmark of the inflammatory or autoimmune state.

As Pollack has shown, all fourth-phase water has a negative electric charge and functions as a crystalline gel-receptive device that can absorb various forms of outside information, energy, and signals.[1] Think of a radio receiver, which absorbs certain frequencies of radio waves and converts them into the sounds we hear through a radio. So the gel—that is, cytoplasm as it exists in a healthy fourth state—serves two functions: It creates the negative field of electrons that form a halo around each cell, and it acts as a receptive device allowing the cell to receive outside information, energy, and signals and convert them into something useful for the life of the organism.

This offers some insight into the role of ATP, which, as we have seen, is typically thought of as the currency of intercellular energy transfer. In the currency model, it is constantly being built, stored, and broken down to provide the energy needed for given cellular functions. I believe it's more accurate to view ATP as playing the same role that heat plays in the formation of gelatin: It binds to certain receptors on the intracellular proteins, which causes a transformational change allowing them to unfold and extend the proteins, so they can bond with water and, when cooled, form a gel with a robust negative charge that provides a protective halo—all without any pumping or outside energy required.

In a series of experiments, Gilbert Ling was able to show that because of the specific physical characteristics of this fourth-state intracellular gel—a meshlike gel structure inside the cell—the cell is precisely configured to "trap" the potassium (in the form of K+) inside the cell and exclude the sodium (in the form of N+). To picture this, imagine a screen on a porch window. For some reason, you want to let small mosquitoes into your porch, but you want to exclude bigger flies. You could create a mesh screen that would be just the right size to let mosquitoes in and exclude flies. This is the same way our intracellular gel works, except that in the case of our cells, the mesh itself actually binds to the potassium inside the cell.

Ling's discovery is a precise, self-sustaining system that uses no outside energy for accomplishing perhaps the most important function of the cell, which is to concentrate potassium inside the cell, while excluding sodium. This explanation provides a much more elegant, simple, sustainable, and economical model than that of the pump, which I find implausible notwithstanding its widespread acceptance.

This model of the mammalian cell allows us to understand common phenomena and molecular events differently. For example, it has been shown that the transcription and translation of DNA into proteins depends on which parts of the DNA are exposed or "unfolded" at a given time. Picture a long strand of DNA that consists of one hundred separate genes. Now imagine that as a result of being exposed to estrogen, which can bind with a site on the intracellular gel, what is needed is to make a hundred copies of gene 43. The estrogen signal subtly changes the structure of the crystalline matrix. The DNA embedded in this matrix changes the way it folds as a result of the change in the matrix in which it is embedded. This change in the folding of the DNA exposes gene 43, which is then transcribed and translated into the protein needed and which was the purpose of the estrogen signal. This changes the environment of the DNA and the protein factories of the cell so that the needed proteins are produced. Because of the nature of the fourth phase, these processes—which we call "life"—proceed with a minimum of energy and a maximum of ease.

Again, this is a seamless, energy-free, sustainable system that allows for life to flow with ease. Signals, in the form of hormones, ions, and nutrients, all create subtle changes in the intracellular matrix, which subtly changes in response to this exposure. A further beauty of this system is that due to the bipolar nature of water and its ability to form virtually unlimited binding sites, the human cell can be receptive to an unlimited number of outside influences. This explains why water is the foundation for life: It has unlimited flexibility and an unlimited ability to bind with outside influences. No pump system or protein-bound membrane can even remotely approximate this inherent ability of water.

This new way of looking at the cell helps us understand the developing field of epigenetics. The conventional model of genetics is that the primary structure—that is, the sequence of base pairs that make up the DNA molecule—is everything. We have a trillion-dollar biotech industry devoted to sequencing DNA and finding out the makeup of our genes. What this new model demonstrates is that, while the DNA sequences that make up our genes are relevant, what is much more important is how and when each DNA sequence will be unmasked or unfolded so it can be copied. This process is what actually determines our health.

In Bruce Lipton's seminal book on epigenetics, *The Biology of Belief*, he showed that even with the most common genetic diseases, the outcomes were often largely determined by epigenetic influences, which might even include an individual's belief system. Let's say on chromosome 11 there is gene 20, and if you make a hundred copies a day of the protein derived from gene 20, you get the symptoms of multiple sclerosis. However, if you only make eighty copies of gene 20 per day, you're fine.

The determinant of the activity of the gene is not the gene itself; that is fixed. The determinant is whether it is exposed or unfolded, signaling the production of protein. This is a function of the crystalline gel, not of the DNA itself. In other words, the gel, not the DNA, determines the outcome. And water crystalline gel, through its almost infinite number of binding sites, is the perfect receptive vehicle, capable of binding with hormones, vitamins, nutrients, sunlight, sound, light, and—I believe—even more subtle energies such as belief and love. All of these influences can be shown to interact with and change the shape of the crystalline gel. This model then gives us an actual physiologic explanation of how our genes are influenced by what we think, feel, and say, and who we are around. Everything in our shared environment has a clear influence on who we are and how we function, even down to the details of how our genes are expressed.

CHAPTER SEVEN

Spatial Orientation, Autism, and Autoimmunity

After I graduated from college and completed a tour of service in the Peace Corps, I grew very interested in and involved with anthroposophy and anthroposophical medicine. I went to medical school, during which time I completed four months of medical apprenticeships at doctors' practices associated with Camphill communities. I lived with a family in the village, participated in the life of the home, including cooking, cleaning, and doing other chores, and spent two days a week working in the village.

The Camphill movement revolutionized the care of developmentally disabled people around the world. Started by a physician named Karl Konig in Scotland who was inspired by Rudolf Steiner, the Camphill movement changed the way disabled people are cared for and participate in community life—from living in often dismal and isolated situations to having opportunities to live fulfilling lives with joy and dignity. Decades later and with Camphill villages all over the world, the communities continue to serve as a model for how humans can live together in a new way.

In Camphill communities, typically between two and ten disabled people—some villages are oriented to adults, others to children—also live in homes with families, along with one to three co-workers or volunteers. During the day, the villagers (the disabled) go either to school, if they are children, or to work, if they are adults. The work might include gardening, animal husbandry, woodworking, bookbinding, or any other skill that someone in the community might possess. Sometimes the villagers work in a café, serving meals from food grown in their gardens to area residents and townspeople. The villagers might choose a single job they prefer or be assigned jobs through which they rotate on a regular basis. When I apprenticed in the villages, I typically worked in the gardens because I knew something about growing food. I was generally assigned a crew of two or three villagers and we all worked under the supervision of one of the staff gardeners, with tasks that included shoveling manure, digging garden beds, planting, weeding, and harvesting.

During this time, I worked with two teenagers, Fred and Paul, who had severe autism. Paul was about fifteen when I met him at a Camphill village in upstate New York. While we were together, Paul would often rock back and forth, twirl sticks, and sing "blah blah" in a variety of melodies. He was strong and could shovel manure and put it in the cart, but he really preferred to be left alone in his own world, so it was hard for me to be too much of a taskmaster. What fascinated me, however, was how much Paul enjoyed weeding and, as far as I ever saw, he never pulled out a garden plant instead of a weed. When I weeded the carrot bed, I found it difficult to distinguish the carrots from the weeds and, especially if I was moving quickly, I often mistook one for the other and mistakenly pulled out tiny carrot seedlings rather than weeds. But Paul easily weeded more quickly than I and with far fewer mistakes. I once asked him how he did it. He responded with the joyous twirl of a stick, a Cheshire Cat grin, and the melodious "blah blah" of a song.

Fred was eighteen when I met him at the same Camphill village in upstate New York. A big, burly guy, he came charging toward me with his arms flapping the first time—and all subsequent times—I met him. He stopped a few feet before plowing into me and asked me something about "Uncle Harry." Honestly, it was terrifying at first, but once I got to know him, it was clear that he would never hurt anyone. Once I completed medical school, I moved to New Hampshire and set up my small family practice in the midst of a thriving anthroposophical community and near the local Camphill village. Fred and Paul both eventually moved to the New Hampshire Camphill village near where I lived and worked as the village doctor for seventeen years.

Once I'd established my practice, I got to know a new villager named Jimmy, who was my age, about thirty at the time. Jimmy was short with a stocky build, a humped back, and a pronounced limp. He had a pressured, quick way of talking and tremendous anxiety, particularly about his own health. But Jimmy loved music and could play numerous instruments, even sight-reading complex musical pieces. The village was a wonderful place for him because, like most Camphill villages, it emphasized and encouraged engagement with the arts as much as possible. I watched Jimmy with his clarinet, and given the score for a new clarinet sonata, he played it perfectly the first time through. The notes were spot-on and the rhythm was impeccable, but it sounded terrible, like it came from a machine that had been programmed to play the notes in rhythm without any conception at all that it was actually a piece of music. No matter how or how often we tried to convey this sense of musicality to Jimmy—because we thought perhaps it would enrich his experience—or even played a recording for him of the same sonata, Jimmy played it the same every time, exactly as he did the first time. He didn't seem to have a way to conceptualize what I meant when I tried to convey the musicality or the feeling of the piece.

Jimmy could do other amazing things. For example, if I took a box of pick-up sticks or building blocks and tossed them on the floor, within seconds, Jimmy would tell me how many sticks or blocks there were. He could also instantaneously tell me the day of the week for any date in the last 2,000 years—somehow it gets complicated around 0 AD.

Jimmy used to like to come to my office, and I always scheduled at least thirty minutes for his visit so we had some time to hang out. He often walked into the exam room and started moaning "Ow" even before I touched him. Sometimes when I examined him, he made all sorts of painful groaning sounds—but with a grin on his face. I asked him if these things were really painful, as no one had reported any injury or problem to me. Looking like a child caught with his hand in the cookie jar, Jimmy admitted that he was "fine, just fine," but that you never know if you're about to be struck dead from a seizure or stroke, or some other malady he'd recently heard or read about. The rest of the time, he peppered me with questions to allay his fears that something was horribly wrong with him. He would seem OK for a while, until he'd come see me again for more aches and pains.

Over the years I got to know Jimmy's mother well, and she confided in me that in spite of taking Jimmy to all the best doctors at Children's Hospital and Mass General in Boston, and to some of the most well-known holistic and alternative practitioners on the East Coast, no one had any idea what to do to help him. Like many parents, she had seen the onset of his symptoms when he was around two. She had also, as was common at that time, been through years of questioning her emotional bond with her child, as well as the all-too-common destruction of the health of their family.

Most Camphill communities are filled with stories: Children who were thought to be well and developing normally begin to develop bizarre symptoms at between fifteen and twenty-four months, often following an adverse reaction to vaccines. Over time, these stories have become more and more common in the population at large, with recent health surveys showing that up to one in thirty-six children is now considered on the autism spectrum.

———

I owe a debt of gratitude to these young autistic people because knowing them enriched my life. And more than anyone, they helped me think in different ways about autism, autoimmune disorders, and vaccines—ways that I hope will prove useful in terms of understanding why so many children are now experiencing these disorders and what we can do to prevent and treat them. In Jimmy's case, conventional medicine probably would have given him a diagnosis of idiopathic autism—meaning the cause is unknown—with developmental delay. But to me this doesn't really explain much. It certainly doesn't give any insight into what caused his condition or how it might be prevented in the future. Nor does it offer much in terms of what his lived experience is like, or how we might interact with him to make it better or as positive as possible.

So what if we approach this from a new direction, a direction in which we let the phenomena of what we are seeing speak for themselves?

Take, for example, Jimmy's unusual relationship to music. Music has at least three distinct components. The first is the series of notes, the second is the rhythm of those notes, and the third is the musicality of the piece. The first two can be described mathematically and are noted in the score. That is: at this point you play this note in this temporal relationship to the notes around it. With the musicality, however, there is nothing to write on the paper. People listening to the music have a clear sense of the musicality, but still it can't be put on paper. One way I think of this is that the musicality lives in the *spaces* between the notes and rhythm. When Jimmy played music, it was as though this spatial world wasn't there for him. Jimmy's other behavior also suggested to me an unusually close connection with the world of numbers and things—I believe this was the reason he could do computer-like calculations almost instantaneously.

In Fred, I saw a variation of this disordered spatial awareness. Autistic people often have difficulty navigating social situations. The connections between people are loaded with spatial significance. When a patient comes to my consultation room, we are typically seated a comfortable distance—about two to four feet—apart. But what if I back my chair up to the corner of the room? Or pull my chair to within six inches of my patient's chair? Even though we are the same two people, wearing the same clothes, having the same conversation, changing the space changes everything. Fred didn't have much awareness of his spatial presence. He violated the personal space of others, often putting his face within inches of the person he was talking with. He also had little awareness of his own personal space, frequently bumping into things and running around as if chasing something, perhaps himself. Paul exhibited many of these same traits—a sense of not knowing where he ended and someone else began, of being in constant motion, particularly with repeated hand flapping, as if on a mission to define his boundaries.

Human beings live within their personal space. Personal space, as written and spoken about by my friend Jaimen McMillan, is the egg-shaped invisible cocoon that envelops each of us. Imagine putting your arms out and your hands together in front of you to make a kind of circle in front of your heart. This is the normal boundary of your personal space. If you watch two expert ballroom dancers, you see a perfect example of how meeting another at this border of personal spaces creates the possibility for beautiful and powerful movement. If the dancers come together too closely, the power and the beauty of the movement are lost.

Consider a boxer. Part of his strategy is to get in position to deliver a blow to his adversary right at the edge of his personal space. Muhammad Ali, in his fight with the more powerful

George Foreman, was able to defeat his opponent by spending the entire fight inside Foreman's personal space, thereby taking away Foreman's power. Watch expert Tai Chi masters and you can almost visually see them manipulate and dance with the boundaries of their personal space. When we are in our best health, we meet the world at the edge of our fully intact personal space. We are able to extend our personal space to the tips of our outstretched arms and joined hands and meet the world at this powerful interface.

When we are ill, our personal space contracts, often shrinking right to the boundary of our skin. We can't help but feel exposed, powerless, and vulnerable. It is as if the world is right in our face and this is a profoundly painful experience. This is the world that an autistic person inhabits. Sometimes she acts this out by literally meeting other people right at the border where their skin ends rather than in the healthy orientation of outstretched hands. This, I argue, is the underlying basis for the loss of social functioning that marks autism. It is the shrinking of personal space, which is essentially the shell that encases, protects, and nourishes us all.

Consider cancer cells for a moment. While there are many ways to describe the abnormalities found in cancer cells, particularly in regard to the DNA and number of chromosomes, one characteristic of solid tumors is that the cells have lost their proper spatial orientation to one another. Within each organ, healthy cells have a healthy distance from one another, which is unique to that organ or tissue. Liver cells have their own spatial orientation and distance from one another; heart cells have another. This gives the organ its characteristic feel and texture and is an important aspect of its function. But with solid cancers, this spatial relationship is lost. The cells are effectively too close to one another; the tissue then becomes too dense and too compacted. It becomes the hard mass we call a tumor.

This is where cell biology and the role of water in cell physiology are crucial. Personal space is essentially an emanation of the collective charges generated at the cellular level. As we have seen in chapter 6, each cell generates a halo of negative charges on its exterior. This makes the cell a charged body capable of carrying out cellular functions. When an uncharged cell falls out of the interlinked community of charged cells, it becomes an "alien" cell unable to participate in, and no longer subject to, the overarching order that coordinates and rules over the community of charged cells and makes it an "organism." The uncharged cell clumps together with other uncharged cells, eventually forming into dysfunctional tissue or, in the extreme, tumorous growth.

As we have seen in chapter 6, while conventional science explains the creation of the cellular charge as a function of the sodium-potassium pump, Ling proved that this pump plays only a trivial role in the distribution of these important ions within and without of the cell. Ling also proved that with no external energy required, this distribution of sodium and potassium is achieved almost entirely through water's capacity for forming a crystalline gel matrix, which due to its characteristic size excludes sodium from its matrix (and thus from the cell) and binds selectively to potassium, thus concentrating potassium within the cell. This separation of sodium and potassium produces the halo of negative charges around each cell, allowing the cell to be an active, healthy working unit.

The individual cells form themselves into tissues, which maintain the cumulative charge of the individual cells, and the tissues form themselves into an organism, which has the cumulative charge of the individual cells and tissues. This becomes our personal space. In other words, our personal space is an emanation of the properties of the fourth-phase water in our organism. One might even call this our "water body" or, to use the words of Rudolf Steiner, our "etheric body." Ancient Greek philosophers described this water body as our "life body," or the source of life and the distinction between a living being and a dead or inanimate substance.

It is our water body that is disturbed by vaccines. And our water body is the seat of the pathology in autism and other autoimmune diseases, each with its own manifestations of the disturbance.

How does this disturbance of our water body come about, and what is the connection with vaccines? I think that our water structure gets disturbed through the introduction of an intracellular toxin that inserts itself into the crystalline gel of our cells and degrades it. This, I believe, is the effect of cellular poisons such as aluminum, mercury/thimerosal, formaldehyde, and other toxic chemicals and metals. By inserting themselves into our intracellular matrix, these substances interfere with the charge-generating ability of the cell.

And because the intracellular matrix determines the expression of the DNA by unfolding and shaping our DNA according to its design, with the introduction of vaccines, we see errors and disturbances in DNA transcription and translation into proteins. Conventional science explains this as a result of the mutations that they say "cause" autism, but they place far too much emphasis on DNA mutations and not enough attention on the thing that actually controls DNA function: our intracellular water matrix. When you combine the cells' failure to generate an adequate charge and errors in DNA translation into proteins, the result is the pathology of our water body.

The other way vaccines disturb the intracellular gel matrix is through chronic inflammation. A cell or tissue that is subject to chronic inflammation becomes heated, which first results in the "dissolving" of the intracellular matrix. After the inflammation has been present for a while, the overly heated cells tend to sclerose, or harden, which is another way the intracellular matrix gets degraded. First the intracellular gels dissolve; then they harden. Both processes create an intracellular matrix that has seen its health compromised.

When our cells and tissues are infected or exposed to toxins, our bodies respond by raising the heat, increasing inflammation, dissolving the gels, and excreting the dissolved invasion through liquid water, which can flow—so they can then rebuild healthier gels. This is the rationale for the increased mucus, stool, urination, and sweat that we see as part of an acute illness. And this is the root of Hippocrates's wisdom when he said, "Give me a fever and I can cure any disease." The fever carries out the detoxification process.

Unfortunately, in an autoimmune disease this liquefaction-based detoxification system never comes to resolution. Either because the toxic exposure is too great, the bombardment of absorbed antigens is too continual, or the vicious circle of cellular breakdown constantly stimulates the production of new antibodies, the process never ends. In many cases, it continues until the eventual destruction of the tissues.

Autism is a special case in which this autoimmune process affects the brain itself. When an otherwise normal, healthy child has a bout of uncontrolled screaming following an MMR vaccine, he is experiencing inflammation of the brain, otherwise known as encephalitis. When a child is exposed to known neuro-toxins such as aluminum or thimerosal (a form of mercury) along with surfactants such as polysorbate 80, which facilitate absorption of toxins through barriers, including the blood-brain barrier, he is experiencing a toxic exposure within the brain that the body is attempting to rid itself of with the inflammatory process of liquefaction. When a child fails to establish a healthy gut microbiome due to antibiotic use, poor diet, and exposure to toxins, she is also establishing conditions for which the body's only recourse is inflammation in an attempt to clear these toxins.

The problem is not just vaccines, however. Glyphosate, also known as Roundup, is also an integral part of this, as Dr. Zach Bush has shown. Dr. Bush found that glyphosate stimulates zonulin production, which opens the gaps in our intestinal wall and blood-brain barrier. This excessive zonulin creates a situation where the blood is exposed to toxins and antigens, which normally would have been unable to traverse the gut wall. Once in the blood, excessive zonulin also facilitates the toxins' passage through the blood-brain barrier, introducing them into the brain, to which the body responds with a liquefying, inflammatory process.

Unfortunately, because glyphosate is on most of the fields on which conventionally grown animals are raised, and gelatin obtained from these animals is the medium on which many of the viruses used to make vaccines are grown, glyphosate is a normal component of most vaccines and much of the food our children are eating. Glyphosate on food opens the gut to toxins; glyphosate in vaccines opens the blood-brain barrier to these toxins.

I believe that in the early part of the twentieth century parents had legitimate fears of losing their children to childhood diseases. Diphtheria, in particular, caused outbreaks of disease that left many children dead. As medical science progressed and scientists discovered the diphtheria toxin, a call to vaccinate against it was a legitimate undertaking and a legitimate medical breakthrough. The problem from the beginning was this: Could a vaccine against the diphtheria toxin be developed that didn't otherwise interfere with a child's immune system or compromise the child's health in another way? My understanding, after years of studying the science behind vaccines, is that a truly safe and effective vaccine has not yet been discovered.

Some of the problems with existing vaccines may never be solvable, and one of the biggest problems is that in order for a child to mount an effective immune response, toxic adjuvants that alter the balance of the immune system must often be used. Vaccines in which adjuvants are not needed, generally because they are developed with live viruses, also carry a risk of an excessive and damaging immune response. These and other problems with vaccines may, in fact, never be solvable. But they must, at the very least, be acknowledged.

The consequence of ignoring these risks—along with ignoring the risk of other substances such as glyphosate that have become pervasive in our lives—is that we've neither eradicated childhood illnesses nor reduced our fear of them. Arguably just the opposite has occurred. While the specific diseases have changed since the days of diphtheria and whooping cough, childhood diseases overall are now more pervasive. What parent today doesn't worry about her child having food allergies, eczema, asthma, ADD/ADHD, learning difficulties, autism, or leukemia? Our communities, hospitals, and schools are filled to the brim with sick and injured children—often suffering from illnesses that barely existed a hundred years ago.

In the next section of this book, I look at three quintessential illnesses against which American children today are commonly vaccinated, the vaccine programs that have arisen around these illnesses, and the flaws of those programs.

PART II

Vaccine Fallacies: Three Case Studies

CHAPTER EIGHT

The Chicken Pox Vaccine: A Case of (Un)intended Consequences

Not long ago, pretty much everyone got chicken pox as a kid. Some of us still bear a scar or two from the pox or even have nostalgic memories of a childhood bout with the intensely itchy and uncomfortable pox—maybe of getting it while on vacation, or the time when all the kids in a family (or neighborhood!) came down with it at once. Parents nursed their kids with oatmeal baths, calamine lotion, wet washcloths, and lots of attention. While nobody loves getting sick, or seeing their children sick, nearly everyone experienced full recovery, and gained lifelong immunity. Many people actually harbor warm memories of being intently cared for—or caring for their own children—and the particular bonding that occurs when one nurses another who is acutely ill.

During my first decade of practice in rural New Hampshire nearly all of my pediatric patients got chicken pox at some point during their childhood. We—that is: me, their parents, and members of the community—thought nothing of it. Over the years, there were hundreds and hundreds of cases of chicken pox among my patients, most of whom I never saw because they were not in any real distress. I can't recall a single adverse outcome or complicated course of the illness. If asked, I might have recommended a spoonful of cod liver oil for the vitamin A, some extra vitamin C, and Rhus tox, a homeopathic remedy derived from poison ivy. Otherwise, I didn't get involved.

So I was shocked when I heard that a chicken pox vaccine was being introduced in 1995. I couldn't imagine the rationale for a vaccine that doesn't even offer lifelong immunity for a basically insignificant illness.[1]

Also known as varicella, chicken pox is caused by infection with the varicella zoster virus (VZV), which is in the herpes family. It is highly contagious; most children will come down with clinical chicken pox on first exposure. After a brief incubation period, most will develop a low-grade fever, congestion, a runny nose, and an itchy, blistery rash that typically lasts about a week, before experiencing a full recovery and immunity for life. While chicken pox is typically more serious in adults, it is rare.

An estimated four million Americans got chicken pox each year prior to introduction of the varicella vaccine and while a small number of those cases led to hospitalization from complications such as infection or dehydration, they resulted in only 100 to 150 deaths, about half of whom were adults.[2] I would never dismiss the grief caused by these extremely rare cases, but it's important to understand that this is a very low rate of mortality. For the vast majority of people, chicken pox is a totally benign disease. Everyone knew this in the early 1990s, so it baffled me then how chicken pox came to be seen—or perhaps marketed—so differently.

And in fact, evidence is mounting that battling acute childhood diseases is protective against a whole host of illnesses later in life. In 2007, the peer-reviewed journal *Atherosclerosis* published a paper that concluded, "Childhood contagious diseases had a protecting effect against coronary heart disease. The risk for acute coronary events decreased significantly with increasing number of childhood contagious diseases."[3] Last year, a large study conducted by researchers at the Baylor College of Medicine and reported in the journal *Cancer Medicine* found a 21 percent reduced risk of developing glioma (a deadly brain cancer) among those who had chicken pox as children.[4] The study, one of the largest to date, looked at 4,533 cases and 4,171 controls collected across five countries. "It provides more of an indication that there is some protective benefit from having the chicken pox," reported Dr. Melissa Bondy, lead researcher, McNair Scholar, and associate director for cancer prevention and population sciences at Baylor. "The link is unlikely to be coincidental."

When I read the medical literature at the time the vaccine was introduced in 1995, the best explanation I encountered to justify the introduction of a vaccine was a reference suggesting that parents would have to take fewer days off work to care for their children. Fewer days off work to care for children may provide short-term relief for overburdened parents, but it also results in lost opportunity to witness, watch, and care for our children as they work through an illness—an experience that builds their trust in us as parents and deepens our understanding of our children and their needs. When we always strike preemptively by overvaccinating, overpathologizing, and overtreating children from a very young age, we forfeit the opportunity to develop a deep understanding of the people we love, and want to know, best. If nursed through an illness, once the child is well, he's felt his parent's presence when it was needed. And the parent has developed experience on which to draw when accompanying him through other "battles"—whether behavioral, emotional, or medical. Wise parents know that it's not our job to orchestrate the world so that our children never encounter any conflict or challenge; it's our job to be present with them, aware, and available, as they make their way through a given experience from which they have the opportunity to grow.

———————

The challenge with chicken pox is that while it nearly always resolves quickly with little complication, the virus remains dormant in the nerve roots and may reemerge later as herpes zoster, also known as shingles. Shingles, which has traditionally occurred in older or immune-compromised patients, causes the eruption of a blistery rash along a single nerve root. While the skin rash itself is uncomfortable, it's the internal irritation along the nerve root that people often describe as intensely painful. And it can last for months, even years. Shingles is an unfortunate, often debilitating, and sometimes chronic complication of having had chicken pox—and one of the more difficult illnesses to cope with. While the most common experience of shingles is a painful chronic condition, by the Centers for Disease Control and Prevention's (CDC) own numbers, shingles also results in approximately ninety-six deaths per year, more or less comparable to the mortality rate of chicken pox prior to introduction of the vaccine.[5]

Luckily, shingles is uncommon in the healthy adult population—or at least it was until everything changed in the mid-1990s with the introduction of the varicella vaccine. In the early 2000s, consequences started to become clear—a massive decrease in cases of chicken pox coupled with a massive increase in the number of cases of shingles. A 2005 study on the incidence of varicella and herpes zoster in Massachusetts concluded: "As varicella vaccine coverage in children increased, the incidence of varicella decreased and the occurrence of herpes zoster increased."[6] According to a 2002 study published in the journal *Vaccine*, "Mass varicella vaccination is expected to cause a major epidemic of herpes-zoster, affecting more than 50% of those aged 10–44 years at the introduction of vaccination."[7] Another study reported that between 1999 and 2003, the chicken pox vaccination rate among children between nineteen and thirty-five months of age increased from 66 percent to 89 percent. Cases of shingles in all age groups (including the elderly) increased by 90 percent. Cases of shingles in people ages twenty-five to forty-four significantly increased by 161 percent.[8]

A 2005 *Vaccine* study concluded, "Under universal varicella vaccination, there has been a vaccine-induced decline in exogenous boosting. We estimate universal varicella vaccination has the impact of an additional 14.6 million herpes-zoster cases among adults under 50 years during a 50 year time span at a substantial cost burden of 4.1 billion U.S. dollars or 80 million dollars annually."[9] In other words, the reason the rate of shingles was lower prior to the introduction of the varicella vaccine in 1995 is that, while people harbored the virus in their nerve roots after recovering from chicken pox and were therefore susceptible to shingles, they were also getting "boosted" through periodic exposure to chicken pox, which protected them from shingles.[10] That experience of caring for an acutely ill child suffering with chicken pox? It was also protecting mom and dad from shingles.

Among the most regrettable consequences of the varicella vaccine is that shingles began striking people at a much younger age—those in their forties and fifties, a population that prior to the chicken pox vaccine had almost complete immunity to shingles. Because shingles only occurs when someone has already had chicken pox, some have argued that people are getting shingles because they fall into the age group of people who weren't vaccinated but aren't getting the protective effect of exogenous boosting because the following generation is vaccinated. The argument goes that shingles will disappear once everyone is vaccinated against varicella and there no longer remains a window of unvaccinated people who got chicken pox as children, still harbor the virus, but don't receive the exogenous boosting of unvaccinated children.

The trouble is that universal vaccination will never eradicate the varicella virus, the vaccine is not as protective or long-lasting as the natural immunity conferred by the disease, and the vaccine is becoming less effective over time as more people are vaccinated. You can get shingles even if you've had the varicella vaccine. In fact, you can get shingles *from* the varicella vaccine: A 2011 study in the *Pediatric Infectious Disease Journal* stated that "varicella vaccination of children has decreased disease incidence, *but introduced the occurrence of herpes zoster from vaccine-type virus.*"[11] (Emphasis added.) The authors further stated that "scientists have made laboratory confirmation that *some vaccinated children are developing shingles from the virus in the vaccine.*"[12] (Emphasis added.)

In a 2013 overview of the US universal varicella vaccination program, researchers concluded that "rather than eliminating varicella in children as promised, routine vaccination against varicella has proven extremely costly and has created continual cycles of treatment and disease."[13]

And so Merck, the maker of the Varivax varicella vaccine, did what any massive pharmaceutical company beholden to its shareholders would do: It released Zostavax, a vaccine for herpes zoster. Since 2006, it has distributed in excess of 36 million doses.[14] And like the varicella vaccine, there's no guarantee of lifelong immunity: "The duration of protection beyond four years after vaccination with Zostavax is unknown," the vaccine's insert states.[15]

While this sequence of events was a boon to shareholders—Merck pulled in $749 million in sales from Zostavax in 2016 alone[16]—it was not such a boon to the unsuspecting public. As research into the newly introduced shingles vaccines emerged, so emerged a familiar pattern of vaccine-induced autoimmune diseases. A 2013 study in the *New England Journal of Medicine* found "a 36% increase in the rate of serious adverse events associated with the herpes zoster vaccine in persons 60 years of age or older (compared to a control group)," concluding that, "the efficacy and safety of the herpes zoster vaccine in the elderly are questionable."[17] A study published two years later found that "compared to the unexposed, patients with zoster vaccination had 2.2 and 2.7 times the odds of developing arthritis and alopecia, respectively."[18]

More recently, Zostavax patients have brought a range of suits against Merck. Marc Bern, who is representing plaintiffs in a 2017 suit that claims Zostavax causes injury and death, said his firm has "thousands of complaints" yet to be filed in Philadelphia, with the injuries running "the gamut from contracting shingles as a result of the vaccine all the way to serious personal injuries such as blindness in one eye, individuals who have serious paralysis in their extremities, brain damage, all the way to death."[19] In the same year, plaintiffs from across the country also brought suit against Merck, claiming that far from preventing shingles, Zostavax *gave* them shingles.[20] If the pharmaceutical giant stumbles, there's another waiting in the wings to take its market share: A 2017 report projected that GlaxoSmithKline's shingles vaccine, Shingrix, will more than double its sales by 2022 to $1.17 billion.[21]

If you think that the CDC (or the American Academy of Pediatrics, AAP) is looking out for you and your child as it adds ever more vaccines to the recommended schedule, you may not realize that Julie Gerberding, director of the CDC for seven years, sidestepped right into a lucrative position as president of Merck's vaccine division when President Obama took office in 2009.[22] Or that more than a dozen senior scientists from within the CDC lodged a formal ethical complaint in 2016 about the organization being unduly influenced by "outside parties and rogue interests."[23] Or that a congressional reform committee reported on rampant conflicts of interest between the CDC and vaccine manufacturers, including the chairman's holding of more than 600 shares of stock in Merck.[24]

Many have argued that an organization that has such close ties to the $30 billion vaccine industry, holds dozens of vaccine patents itself, and disseminates much of the "scientific" information coming out about vaccines—which then makes its way into Big Pharma's industry-funded mainstream media outlets—should not have the power to both set the vaccine schedule for US children—a schedule children must either follow or receive an exemption from in order to attend school or most daycares —and oversee vaccine safety.

The question all this leaves me with is this: Did those who developed and aggressively lobbied for the introduction of the varicella vaccine know that a mass vaccination against chicken pox would result in an epidemic of shingles? If they did—and anticipated that it would also open a market for a shingles vaccine —it's unspeakable. If, on the other hand, the shingles outbreak is a consequence nobody predicted or took seriously, that's almost worse, because it suggests that either the experts and institutions we're supposed to trust don't understand what the risks are or what the consequences of vaccination may ultimately be, or they downplay those risks and consequences so significantly that they move forward with questionable vaccination programs regardless.

CHAPTER NINE

The Polio Vaccine: A Case of False Cause

Any book claiming that vaccines have caused or contributed to the explosion of chronic diseases—especially chronic autoimmune diseases in children—must confront many questions about the role vaccines might play in reducing the death, disability, misery, and fear caused by outbreaks of epidemic diseases. No disease in modern history has gripped the country the way polio did in the early and middle decades of the twentieth century. Horrific images of crippled children, adults immobilized in iron lungs, and Franklin Delano Roosevelt leading the country into war from the confines of a wheelchair hold sway in the mind of anyone who lived through it—and in the public imagination to this day. Such was the fear that when Jonas Salk's double-blind vaccine field trial was announced in 1953, the parents of 1.8 million kids rushed to sign them up for the largest medical experiment in the history of the country. When the results were announced a year later—that the vaccine was reportedly safe and 80 to 90 percent effective— it marked a massive turning point, as Americans everywhere breathed a huge sigh of relief and put their faith in the power of vaccines to end human suffering.

It's an incredible story—a modern medical miracle, one that inspired massive eradication initiatives throughout the world, celebrated the triumph of modern science, and ushered in a whole new era of fighting pathogenic disease through the development of vaccines. But what if it's wrong?

According to conventional medical wisdom, poliomyelitis (polio, for short) is a highly contagious infectious disease caused by the poliovirus. The poliovirus is an enterovirus, meaning that it initially infects the enteric, or intestinal, tract. The majority of people who are infected with the poliovirus will have no symptoms; one in four will have flulike symptoms that pass in a few days.[1] And a small number of people infected with the poliovirus will develop paralytic poliomyelitis when the virus gains access to the bloodstream and infects the anterior horn cells of the spinal column—the cells through which our motor neurons pass. In severe cases, the resulting motor dysfunction can include paralysis of the diaphragm, leading to respiratory failure and death—an outcome that led to the development of the iron lung.

Before the vaccine was introduced in early 1955, the predominant public health response to the growing epidemic was to advise people to avoid swimming pools, ponds, lakes, water fountains, and potentially tainted foods because—like other enteroviruses that gain access to the body through the GI tract— the poliovirus is water- or food-borne; that is, the virus is present in an infected person's fecal matter and passes to someone else through fecal-oral transmission on contaminated food or drink. Oral-oral transmission, such as through saliva, on contaminated food or drink, was also possible, but less common.

This is the accepted explanation for the epidemiological phenomenon that led to the twentieth-century polio epidemic in the United States. Some aspects of this explanation are correct, which is part of what makes it so pernicious. In fact, the story is so entrenched that people rarely think to question it, something we must do if we're going to identify the real culprit in the polio epidemic and take measures to ensure that nothing like it ever happens again. The poliovirus *is* an enterovirus and the vaccine *does* create antibodies against it. But other aspects of this explanation are wildly incomplete, or even flat-out wrong. The vaccine did not end the epidemic and the virus was not responsible for it.

How can I draw such a radical conclusion—one completely at odds with everything we think we know about polio? For one thing, a lot of the polio story just doesn't add up. It fails to answer a number of crucial questions, including the one raised by figure 9.1.

Why did paralytic polio make such a sudden and dramatic appearance in the United States in the years between 1916 and 1918? Why were there almost no cases of paralytic polio recorded or described in the medical literature before 1900?

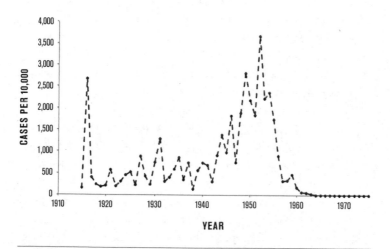

Figure 9.1. The Incidence of Poliomyelitis in the United States 1915–1975. *Source: Dan Olmsted, "The Age of Polio Series: Explosion." Age of Autism: Daily Web Newspaper of Autism Epidemic, 2016. Courtesy of Mark Blaxill.*

Did the virus simply not exist before then? Or did it undergo some sort of mutation that changed it from the source of a common and harmless viral infection into the cause of deadly paralytic polio in 1916? If so, how and why did that happen? We see from figure 9.1 that within a couple of years, the incidence of polio declined. There's no clear reason for this.

If the 1916 outbreak had been the result of a sudden emergence of a harmless virus that mutated into a serious pathogen, we would have seen an explosion of cases as it affected more and more people with no prior exposure. Yet this is not at all what we saw. There were fluctuations in incidence over the years, but nothing like the millions of cases one would expect from a population encountering a new pathogenic virus for the first time.

After a few decades of ups and downs, there was another explosion of polio cases in the late 1940s continuing through the 1950s to its peak at 60,000 in 1952. Introduction of the vaccine in 1955 seemed to coincide perfectly with an almost instantaneous decline, which continued until 1979, when the disease was declared eradicated in the United States. But we still have no explanation for why polio arose so suddenly, seemingly out of nowhere, and the introduction of the vaccine is not the only plausible explanation for why cases dropped off so suddenly. Nor does it explain the curious distribution of cases.

If you look at a map showing the distribution of cases of paralytic polio in the years between 1916 and 1920, it presents an odd pattern for a viral disease. Why were cases of paralytic polio initially clustered around Coney Island, so much so that for years the beaches were virtually deserted? Soon polio appeared in other cities along the East Coast, such as Boston, Philadelphia, and Baltimore; cases were concentrated in large urban centers, rarely in inland towns or rural areas. They occurred largely in big cities, always in neighborhoods close to the sea, with a majority of the victims having some connection with a neighborhood candy store.[2]

Over the next few summers, there was a lot of public discussion about possible reasons for this peculiar distribution. At that time in the United States, pharmaceutical-based medicine was in its infancy and most health practitioners had at least a minimal connection with the role of diet, fresh air, exercise, and a healthy living environment in the health of their patients and community. The disease distribution led to a lot of speculation about the despicable state of the waste treatment in big cities and children being forced to drink "swill milk" from diseased cows fed industrial waste in big-city pens. It is possible, even likely, that poor urban sanitation and industrial waste contributed to the spread of polio, but American cities had been cesspools of disease and despair for decades without polio showing up. Something new and different was happening around 1916.

Neither of these explanations sits well. They're too speculative. Too random. And there are more persuasive explanations for the sudden rise, the curious distribution of cases, and even the sudden decline. To understand, we need to look at other unprecedented events in the years around 1916.

Dan Olmsted was an investigative journalist, former senior editor for United Press International (UPI), assistant national editor at *USA Today*, and one of two journalists who reported on devastating mental health implications of use of the antimalarial drug mefloquine among US service members. Following a series of articles on autism—in which he noted the near complete absence of autism among the Amish—Olmsted left UPI to cofound the *Age of Autism* with Mark Blaxill, Kim Rossi, and J.B. Handley, where he and Blaxill conducted two brilliant investigations into the cause of the twentieth-century polio epidemic, linking it to widespread agricultural use of neurotoxins, including arsenite of soda and DDT.[3]

Many people have made a connection between sugar and these early outbreaks, and the correlation didn't escape investigators or officials at the time either. There were a number of public health and media announcements warning parents not only about bathing sites and beaches, but also about consumption of sugar and sugary foods. Of course, sugar was not new to the American diet; nor was swimming at public beaches. What was new during those years had to do with the sugar coming into the United States, which was mostly grown in Hawaii or Cuba and shipped to refining factories along the East Coast, including one right off Coney Island.[4]

Growing sugarcane can be a nasty business. It depletes soil of its nutrients and doesn't compete well with weeds; weeds on a cane plantation are abundant and prolific. The sharp leaves of the sugarcane cut laborers during weeding and harvest, making the work dangerous, arduous, slow, and subject to frequent labor strikes. During the early years of the twentieth century, the industry was in crisis, as many big Hawaiian cane growers went out of business and others struggled desperately to improve their profit margins.[5]

Then, in the summer of 1913, a Hawaiian plantation owner named Charles Eckhart came up with a solution, literally. His solution was to spray the sugarcane fields with arsenite of soda, a particularly potent form of arsenic. This revolutionary approach, coming at a time when little was known about herbicides and toxicity, seemed miraculous because the arsenic killed the weeds but seemed to leave the cane plants unaffected. Arsenite of soda allowed a drastic reduction in workforce, huge savings, fewer injuries, and higher profits.[6]

The only problem, though not recognized at that time, is that arsenic and, in particular, the arsenite of soda used in the sugarcane fields are not only toxic to tropical weeds, but also highly toxic to fish and other sea mammals, insects, and wildlife in general. And, more relevant for our story, arsenic is specifically toxic to the anterior horn cells of the spinal column. It also creates a strong inflammatory response in the gastrointestinal tract, which often results in thinning of the villous brush border of the intestines.[7] When the villi are damaged, the gut wall becomes leaky, and toxins and pathogens that usually stay within the GI tract gain access to the bloodstream.

What about the first recorded cases of polio in Europe, which occurred in Sweden in 1887, and the polio outbreak in Vermont that occurred just a few years later?[8] Around 1873, the first arsenic-based insecticide was released in Germany for general use in combating the gypsy moth. A year later, the first DDT-type organophosphate insecticide was released, also in Germany, for agricultural use. Both of these products found their way into general use. And Vermont's polio outbreak coincided with the release and widespread use of a lead arsenate spray to control gypsy moths.[9]

What about the apparent absence of polio in animals? Humans are purportedly the only known natural hosts in the animal world (although monkeys have long been experimentally infected with the poliovirus for research purposes). In the 1890s, however, cows in Vermont mysteriously began experiencing acute onset of paralytic disease. The cause was traced back to lead arsenate used to kill gypsy moths, the discontinuation of which led to the end of the acute paralytic disease in the cows.

Researchers at that time were struggling to prove the poliovirus–paralytic polio connection. According to Koch's postulates for proving the cause of a transmittable disease, one must be able to take some bodily fluids from a person (or animal) with a known disease, introduce this into a different person (or animal), and create the identical disease. Researchers remained unable to prove Koch's postulates for a transmissible cause of polio.

In 1908, Austrian physicians Karl Landsteiner and Erwin Popper conducted an experiment in which they drew fluid from the spinal cord of a deceased nine-year-old boy who had been paralyzed and died from complications of what was assumed to be polio. According to a report for *The Vaccine Reaction*, they then filtered "preparations" from this fluid and injected it into the brains of two monkeys. One monkey died and the other was left paralyzed in its legs. When Landsteiner and Popper later dissected the brains of the monkeys, they found that the damaged brain tissue looked similar to the damaged brain tissue of infants diagnosed with infantile paralysis. This experiment is considered the first time scientists isolated the poliovirus and proof of its infectious nature, but still it failed to meet Koch's postulates for infectious disease and was roundly criticized by many, including polio research pioneer and bacteriologist Claus W. Jungeblut, MD, and John Polanyi, PhD, who earned the Nobel Prize in chemistry in 1986.[10]

The conclusion from the experiment was that the preparations taken from the boy (assumed to have had a viral infection) and injected into the monkeys contained a virus that caused paralysis because one of the monkeys showed symptoms of paralysis. That "invisible virus," which Landsteiner and Popper believed they had "isolated," is what has come to be known as the poliovirus.

But what exactly was in the preparations from the boy's spinal cord fluid? What was in the preparations that killed one of the monkeys and paralyzed the other? Was it the poliovirus or could something else have killed and paralyzed the monkeys? This is a critical question, particularly given that the CDC states: "Poliovirus only infects humans."[11]

Prior to injecting the preparations into the brains of the monkeys, Landsteiner and Popper had made the monkeys drink the preparations. The monkeys were not harmed by them. No paralysis. Landsteiner and Popper also injected the preparations into one of the limbs of each monkey. No apparent harm to the animals. No paralysis. The harm occurred only after the preparations were injected directly into their brains.

Is it possible that the death of one of the monkeys and the paralysis of the other monkey were not caused by the virus that came to be known as the poliovirus? The monkeys' brains were injected with foreign cellular tissue, unfiltered toxins from whatever plagued the nine-year-old boy. The tissue probably contained any number of viruses and bacteria. How could Landsteiner and Popper definitively conclude it was one specific virus that killed one monkey and paralyzed the other? Could the large syringe itself that they used have caused serious nerve damage or internal bleeding?

After World War I, the use of arsenic for agricultural purposes became more widespread and episodic outbreaks of polio continued to spread. And, as more of the sugar manufacturers used arsenite of soda on their cane fields, more and more of the sugar coming into the United States was contaminated.

Then, after a few decades of relative decline and stability, came another onslaught of polio cases in the mid- to late 1940s. At that time, there was significant dissent from the theory that this was all due to simply more viral infections, a theory that was established from one tenuous study of injecting poliovirus into the brains of monkeys. Nothing had changed in the virus, so why was it suddenly causing more disease?

One interesting theory as to the dramatic increase in cases of paralytic polio seen in the mid-1940s was that this was the time that the mass vaccination program for the diphtheria, pertussis, and tetanus (DPT) vaccine was introduced. While there are few studies that prove a conclusive link between mass vaccination and the increase in paralytic polio, the connection is plausible enough that vaccine manufacturers routinely state in package inserts not to use certain vaccines in the event of an outbreak of poliomyelitis. This is not unlike the study that examines giving the DPT vaccine to children in Guinea-Bissau, which showed that cases of diphtheria, pertussis, and tetanus decreased in the vaccinated population, but having received the DPT was associated with a higher overall mortality from other causes.[12] Perhaps the same phenomenon is at work here: Introduction of mass vaccination against DPT sufficiently weakened the immune system to make recipients more susceptible to the symptoms we associate with paralytic polio.

In the 1940s, a Connecticut physician named Dr. Morton Biskind had grown concerned after seeing a rise of degenerative disease among his patients. "In the US, the incidence of polio has been increasing prior to 1945 at a constant rate, but its epidemiologic characteristics remain unchanged," he noted. "Beginning in 1946 the rate of increase more than doubled."[13]

Like many others at the time, Biskind began to suggest a relationship between paralysis that was typically attributed to polio and the introduction of DDT. First synthesized in 1874, DDT was introduced commercially in the United States in the 1940s for agricultural and general insecticidal use. Many of us who were kids at that time raced after the truck as it drove down our neighborhood streets spraying DDT. I still have vivid memories of following the truck on my bike amid a cloud of sweet-smelling gas as it went back and forth across our neighborhood ball field. The spraying was a monthly event during summer months, the time of the year when cases of paralytic polio surfaced.

It was well-known even at that time that DDT works by interfering with the central nervous system and it has a specific affinity for the anterior horn cells of the spine. DDT is absorbed through the skin, through food, and through the mucous membranes and has been linked to paralytic disease in animals since the beginning of the twentieth century. In the late 1940s and early 1950s, many researchers began drawing a connection between the widespread use of DDT and the symptoms attributed to paralytic polio. According to Olmsted and Blaxill, "In 1949 . . . Drs. Morton S. Biskind and Irving Bieber published 'DDT Poisoning – A New Symptom With Neuropsychiatric Manifestations' in the *American Journal of Psychotherapy.* 'By far the most disturbing of all the manifestations are the subjective reactions and the extreme muscular weakness,' they reported."[14] In the same year, Daniel Dresden published *Physiological Investigations Into the Action of DDT*, linking DDT poisoning and polio-like symptoms.[15]

In 1952, Dr. Ralph Scoby testified in front of the US House subcommittee investigating polio, asserting that "polio is classic poisoning."[16] And in 1953, Dr. Biskind published a paper in the *American Journal of Digestive Diseases* that issued this damning conclusion: "Central Nervous System diseases such as polio are actually the physiological and symptomatic manifestations of the ongoing government and industry sponsored inundation of the world's populace with central nervous system poisons."[17] When Dr. Biskind testified a year later before the House committee investigating the rise of polio, he said: "It is known that DDT poisoning produces a condition that may be easily mistaken for polio in an epidemic, but also being a nerve poison itself, may damage cells in the spinal cord and this increases susceptibility to the virus."[18] Indeed, there was a

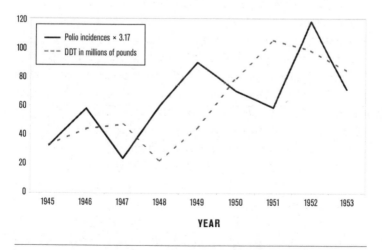

Figure 9.2. Polio Incidence and DDT Production in the United States 1945–1953. *Source: Jim West, "Everything You Learned About the Cause of Polio Is Wrong," Green Med Info, August 21, 2015.*

great deal of overlap between incidence of polio and DDT production. (See figure 9.2.)

An investigation into a 1958 polio outbreak in Detroit showed that only 51 percent of the affected patients tested positive for the virus. What about the other 49 percent, who were diagnosed with paralytic polio but had no evidence of exposure to the causative agent?[19] Again, this statistic violates Koch's postulates, which guide researchers and physicians toward the cause of an infectious disease. There should not be a single case of paralytic polio in people with no exposure to the virus, let alone nearly half of those diagnosed. One must look for another cause for the epidemic.

The end of the polio epidemic in the early 1960s is almost always attributed to the introduction of the Salk vaccine, followed by the Sabin vaccine, which was—ironically—administered via a white sugar cube. There's a correlation, to be sure, between the introduction of the vaccine and the end of the polio epidemic, but, as all scientists should know, correlation does not equal causation. And there's another correlation between the introduction of the vaccine and the end of the polio epidemic: the phasing out, at least in the United States, of DDT; it was, for decades, still shipped overseas, particularly to poorer countries, which then began to see their own polio outbreaks. Around 1964, when the last of the polio epidemics occurred, DDT use had already been severely curtailed in the United States. As we know, it was not the end of the chemical era, but it was the end of an era of chemicals that target the anterior horn cells of our spinal column, bringing about symptoms that are attributed to a common enterovirus within the human gut ecosystem.

The poliovirus has been part of our normal gut ecology for millennia without causing significant disease, certainly without causing epidemics like those the United States saw during the early- and mid-twentieth century. There is no evidence that the virus mutated in a way that would account for new virulence. And, in fact, when outbreaks were investigated, up to half of the victims had no evidence of any infection at all with any poliovirus.

When all is said and done, it is clear that polio is not simply the case of a dangerous virus we finally subdued. While it is possible that the virus is a co-factor in producing what we call paralytic polio, the main etiological agents are the toxins. Without the toxic exposures I outlined, there would have been no polio epidemics, and the massive push toward vaccines against all childhood illness may never have gotten the momentum it did. This is why it is so important, even now, to thoroughly investigate all of the factors involved in the disease we call polio.

CHAPTER TEN

The Measles Vaccine:
A Case of Oversimplification

Compared to polio, measles presents a totally different picture of the role of infectious diseases in sickness and health. As we have seen, polio is actually not an infectious disease at all; rather it is the result of specific poisons affecting distinct areas of our nervous system. As a result, concerns about spreading infection and herd immunity are not—or should not be—a significant part of the debate about polio. With measles, on the other hand, we have perhaps *the* classic infectious childhood illness, one that is currently provoking almost hysterical reactions from public health officials and worried parents. Let's take a step back and examine the history of measles and see what we can learn about this quintessential childhood illness.

I say "quintessential childhood illness" because when Rudolf Steiner described a child's stages of development, he pointed out that all children need to go through certain acute inflammatory illnesses in order to develop a harmonious and healthy body. In Steiner's cosmology, human beings have four distinct yet interpenetrating "bodies," each of which needs to be "born," or perhaps liberated, at the correct time. This birth or liberation is often facilitated by a "typical" acute inflammatory illness of childhood, usually accompanied by fever and often a rash. It is as a result of going through and overcoming an illness that the child gains mastery of his overall physical body as well as his unique destiny. The four bodies and examples of the kinds of illnesses that may accompany and facilitate their liberation in the child's growth and development are as follows:

Birth of the physical/mineral body—first year of life—
  whooping cough
Birth of the water body—usually ages 4 to 7—measles
Birth of the air body—usually ages 10 to 14—scarlet fever
Birth of the warmth body—usually ages 18 to 21—
  mononucleosis

Needless to say, growing children are subject to a much greater variety of acute inflammatory illnesses, fevers, and rashes than the four mentioned above. Croup, chicken pox, impetigo, German measles, and many others may "pinch-hit" for the above four, and any such illness may occur relatively long before or after the above-stated ages.

The birth/liberation of a child's three "higher" bodies (water, air, and warmth) can be incremental and is a very individualized and variable living process that each child manifests differently. The important point is that parents and physicians need to develop a healthy sensitivity and respect for the perhaps counterintuitive fact that acute inflammations with fevers, mucus, or rashes are healthy rites of passage in childhood development. Children who are supported to work through these healing crises are invariably healthier and more resilient than children in whom these inflammatory crises have been suppressed with vaccines, antibiotics, and anti-inflammatory drugs.

Every physician knows that in severe cases antibiotics can be life-saving, nevertheless it is an acknowledged fact of modern medicine that antibiotics are very often prescribed unnecessarily.

***

In this chapter we will take up the role of measles in helping the child gain mastery of the all-important watery, or fluid, realm of their being. This is highly relevant in terms of an individual's future health: Research shows that children who successfully go through measles at the usual ages (four to seven years old) have less heart disease, arthritis, allergies, autoimmune diseases, and overall better health than those who never get measles.[1] Children need to undertake the struggle to make their body their own; measles is one vehicle for this to happen.

Measles is an acute infectious disease caused by an enveloped, single-stranded RNA virus of the *Paramyxoviridae* family. People with measles are highly contagious for four days prior to the onset of the rash and for the first four days of the rash, and up to 90 percent of nonimmune children exposed to another child with measles will catch the disease. Transmission is airborne, primarily from being around children with measles who are coughing or sneezing. The entire illness usually consists of a high fever, cough, rash, congestion, and the pathognomonic (disease-defining) Koplik spots inside the cheeks of the child. Complications of measles include ear infections, pneumonia, and, rarely, encephalitis (inflammation of the brain). The congestion that accompanies a measles infection is more profuse than with practically any other acute illness. Often, it seems as if the child is pouring out gallons of thick mucus from all of his respiratory passages. The rash can also be intense, although generally it is only mildly to moderately itchy.

The most significant aspect in the history of measles is that it was among the many infectious diseases that European settlers brought to the New World that devastated Native American populations. Because settlers brought so many infectious diseases, it's hard to pinpoint the most destructive ones—other than smallpox, which we know was the deadliest, in part because settlers waged biological warfare with it. Some historians estimate that infectious diseases were responsible for killing as many as twenty million people, or up to 95 percent of the Native American population.[2] While some people point to this as an argument for vaccination, the opposite is actually true: The devastation is a cautionary tale about what can happen when people have no prior exposure to an infectious disease—precisely the goal of vaccination-based eradication efforts. We are much, much safer with some exposure to infectious agents. And the course of a measles infection, in particular, offers us crucial insight into why Native Americans were susceptible and why our current vaccine policy is so dangerous.

As I described in chapter 3, we have two immune systems: a cell-mediated system and a humoral system. When we are confronted with an infectious agent (usually a virus or bacteria) to which we have no prior exposure, it enters our body and sets up residence in the cells it has an affinity for. With measles, it's typically the epithelial cells that line our respiratory passages. The infected cells then must be eliminated—the job of the cell-mediated immune system. Calling forth its cadre of white blood cells, cytotoxic chemicals, and enzymes, the cell-mediated immune system dissolves the structure of the cell, liquefying it so it can be mobilized to flow outward. This process gives rise to the profuse mucus discharge seen in children with measles. This cell-mediated cleansing persists for seven to twelve days, after which most cases resolve.

Within about six weeks, the humoral immune system finishes making its antibodies to a protein specific to the virus. The function of the antibodies, specifically made in response to each individual viral infection, is to tag the incoming virus if it is ever encountered again. By tagging and neutralizing the virus with antibodies, the cell-mediated immune system never needs to get involved and the individual will typically never again get sick from the measles virus.

During the first year of life, a child's immune system is not well developed and she is at the highest risk for a complicated course with measles. However, since most mothers, until recently, had measles as children, they harbor the antibodies. When a mother nurses her child for the first one to three years of life, these antibodies pass through the breast milk and protect the child. This is known as passive immunity. In this way, young children are protected until they are old enough to successfully navigate a course of measles and also develop antibodies that will protect them from getting measles as adults—the other time when measles infection can have devastating consequences. This natural protection was so sound that there were almost no serious complications from measles infections in the decade prior to the introduction of the vaccine (figure 10.1).

If this is the case, why then was measles so devastating to Native Americans when settlers brought it from Europe? Because there was no prior exposure in the Native American population, nobody had humoral immunity. Everyone was susceptible, including adults, the elderly, and babies (because

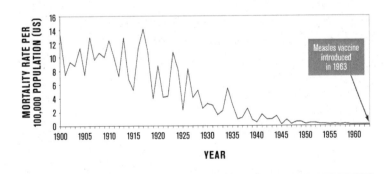

Figure 10.1. Decline in Measles Mortality 1900–1963. *Source: Physicians for Informed Consent, "Disease Information Statement, Measles: What Parents Need to Know," updated December 2017.*

nursing mothers had no protective antibodies to transmit): It was a perfect storm of susceptibility leading to catastrophic outcomes. The majority of Native Americans who died from measles were the very young or the elderly. After the initial encounter, adults were protected and babies received passive antibodies from their mothers—making measles a childhood illness in Native American populations, as it was in Europe. Within a short time the devastation from measles ceased.

What many people don't realize is that by the time the measles vaccine was introduced in 1963, it had ceased to be a public health threat in the United States. Mortality from measles had already declined 98.5 percent from 13.3 per 100,000 to 0.2 per 100,000, due to improvements in living conditions, nutrition, and medical care, according to Physicians for Informed Consent (see figure 10.1).[3] In the decades prior to the introduction of the vaccine, parents had such a casual attitude about it that they frequently held measles parties to ensure their children's exposure. Doctors discovered that giving their young measles patients adequate vitamin A in the form of cod liver oil was sufficient to protect them from complications. And it was understood that the only people who were really at risk were the very young and the elderly and that both demographics could be protected by exposure at the appropriate time. Then, less than ten years after the polio vaccine was introduced, the measles vaccine came along and changed the way we think about measles.

A few years later, a paper published in the medical literature illustrated to public health officials and pediatricians a surprising story about immunity to measles. It described the case of a child born with the genetic inability to make antibodies; that is, he was born without a humoral immune system, but his cell-mediated immunity was normal, so when he contracted measles, the infection progressed in the normal way. Researchers predicted that because the child was unable to make antibodies, he would contract measles infections over and over. While researchers couldn't deliberately expose the child to measles to test their hypothesis, they could follow the child over the course of a few decades. To their amazement, despite repeated exposure, he never contracted measles again.[4] While it's possible he wasn't ever again exposed to measles, I think the better explanation is that our understanding of humoral immunity is flawed. The cell-mediated immune system does, in fact, play a role in remembering and preventing repeat infections and, in a pinch, it can entirely serve this function. In other words, a cell-mediated reaction is sometimes sufficient to confer lifelong immunity.

This case is significant because when a child is vaccinated—when she's injected with an attenuated virus and various neurotoxic adjuvants—she loses the benefit of any cell-mediated response and what we see is primarily a humoral response.

Vaccine manufacturers, pediatricians, public health officials, and the media assure us that the immunity conferred by a vaccine is identical to the immunity conferred by illness, but with a vaccine, there is limited cell-mediated response. With the measles vaccine, the immunity isn't lifelong and confers none of the immunological benefits of fighting the disease.

Fifteen years after a mass vaccination program got under way, young adults started to get the measles again. Because vaccine-based immunity isn't lifelong, adults and the elderly were once again susceptible, and because the antibodies did not persist into adulthood, unlike their persistence in every case of natural measles, nursing mothers no longer had antibodies to pass on to their children. So people started, and have continued, to get boosters, even though there's no evidence to support the notion that boosters will lead to lifelong immunity either. The measles vaccine program has turned us, immunologically speaking, into Native Americans before they encountered Europeans, with the very old and the very young highly susceptible to devastating infection.

It's no wonder public health officials are so worried about outbreaks. They have no plausible way to protect the elderly or young children. Mothers no longer have antibodies to pass to their nursing children and it is too dangerous to repeatedly vaccinate adults against measles because they're too susceptible to complications from the vaccine. We are in a precarious and unnecessary situation because we chose to interfere with a population that had already effectively neutralized measles.

Nephrotic syndrome is a relatively rare autoimmune disease in which, for unknown reasons, the body makes antibodies to its own kidneys. These antibodies create an inflammatory reaction in the basement membrane of the kidney, causing the kidneys to leak protein into the urine. Protein levels in the blood, and then in the cells, drop. This impacts the cell's ability to maintain proper structure inside the cell, leading to the liquefaction of cytoplasm and "dead" water, or edema. Prior to the introduction of the measles vaccine, if a child with nephrotic syndrome contracted measles, the nephrotic syndrome usually went into remission and never returned. Autoimmune diseases are largely cases of cell-mediated immune system suppression and humoral immune system activation; nephrotic syndrome is a classic example of this and also specifically involves a disturbance in how the child handles the structuring of their water. Measles infection heals both of these.

Every measles infection involves an intense activation of the cell-mediated immune system. This rebalances our cell-mediated and humoral immune response. And, as Steiner suggested, measles allows the child to gain mastery over her water body, or how she handles fluids. This ability to manage fluids is impaired in nephrotic syndrome, and natural measles infection repairs this ability. It is only natural, then, that when the measles vaccine was introduced, it was given to patients with nephrotic syndrome with the expectation that, since the vaccine gives an identical immunologic response as the natural illness, it, too, would cure nephrotic syndrome. But nothing happened: The measles vaccine confers no benefit for a child with nephrotic syndrome. Without the actual illness, without the activation of the cell-mediated immunity, without the struggle the child undergoes to overcome and heal from measles, there is no protection. Vaccination can never confer identical immunity to that which is gained from experiencing an acute illness.

While measles can be devastating, once natural immunity exists across a population, it ceases to be a public health issue. Even the CDC's own statistics on the history of measles infection in the United States show this. Today, however, rather than allowing our children to go through an illness that can confer lifelong protection against subsequent exposure as well as a separate chronic disease (nephrotic syndrome), we inject them with neurotoxins that compromise their immune response. As we have seen, when a child contracts measles, he has an intense involvement and restructuring of his ability to handle water. From a health perspective, there is no more fundamental "skill" for a human being to have than the ability to properly structure water. When the opportunity to develop this skill is denied, worse diseases develop. The trade-off we see in the case of measles—between the previous acute, protection-conferring childhood disease and the current chronic public health disaster—exemplifies the story of pediatric medicine over the last four decades.

PART III

Treatment and Recovery

CHAPTER ELEVEN

Basic Autoimmune Treatment Protocol for Children and Adults

T reatment of any disease must follow directly from an understanding of how the disease arose in the body. If our understanding of the root cause, or causes, is incorrect, our treatment will be, too. If we have a strong understanding of the root cause, we're far more likely to be able to successfully treat or even cure the disease. There are many different ways to practice medicine—our country happens to be in the grip of an intensely profit-driven allopathic way of practicing it at the moment—and it is the investigation and elucidation of the root cause that distinguish one from another.

Sometimes the root cause of a disease, or of a poor outcome, lies not in the patient's body, but in the social, cultural, or economic context in which he lives. If we wanted to understand why a dolphin was sick, we would naturally be interested in the quality of the water in which she lives. Recently a friend of mine who is a veterinarian told me that if cows eat high brix pasture (brix is a marker of the nutrient content of plant material), they never get sick. All living organisms are a complex mixture of inheritance, which we sometimes overly simplify with the word *genetics*, and environment.

Severe vitamin A deficiency is strongly associated with complications or poor outcomes in measles infections. Diets deficient in vitamin A are almost always the result of extreme poverty, often when people have been forcibly displaced from land or a traditional way of life. One approach to reducing complications and poor outcomes—and I'd argue that it's a superficial approach—is to give children measles vaccines. This may affect the mortality rate from measles, which makes the optics and the metrics of vaccination look favorable, but it doesn't ultimately improve the overall health or the lives of children living in extreme poverty. On the contrary, it obscures the root cause and allows medical professionals to tell themselves that they are saving the lives of children, when in fact they are not. It's an approach that serves the psychological needs of adults, not the very real physical needs of children.

In fact, in 1981, researchers conducted a study in an urban region of Guinea-Bissau in which they offered the diphtheria-tetanus-pertussis (DTP) vaccine and the oral polio vaccine (OPV) during three-month checkups to children between the ages of three months and five months. The researchers found that among infants who received the DTP vaccine, there was decreased incidence of death from the diseases for which they were vaccinated, but an increase in overall mortality rate.[1] This was a ground-breaking study that should have served as a clarion call to the entire medical profession and vaccine industry that vaccines should, at least, be studied in this kind of systemic way, but the powers that be have not even bothered to criticize the study, choosing to instead ignore it completely.

A better way to address vitamin A deficiency is to ensure that the patient has a diet with an adequate supply of fats from animals that are pasture-fed or raised on fresh grass or seafoods. Vitamin A is the transformed form of beta-carotene, which is found in many brightly colored vegetables such as carrots and winter squash, but to be effective, the beta-carotene needs to be enzymatically cleaved to form the active vitamin A molecule. This active form of vitamin A, which is effective in the treatment of a wide variety of viral diseases, is found in abundance in the butter or fat of grass-fed cows, the yolks of pasture-raised chickens, wild fish, and other similar animal products. Children, until about the age of twelve, have less of the enzyme needed for the breakdown of beta-carotene into vitamin A. This is why it is crucial, particularly in the prevention of viral diseases, that they have adequate vitamin A stores obtained from the daily consumption of properly raised animal fat. The backup source, used for centuries, is cod liver oil, also a rich source of vitamin A.

Having a poor outcome from measles is a symptom of social displacement, cultural breakdown, and malnutrition. These are difficult issues to address—it is easier to manufacture and administer a vaccine—but these issues must be addressed if we are to truly have a positive impact on the lives of children affected by them.

With that said, when it comes to autoimmune diseases, causes can sometimes be synergistic or beyond an individual's control, such as the case of glyphosate exposure. Medicine, therefore, must be realistic: We must agitate for the complete removal of glyphosate from our ecosystem and at the same time propose a treatment strategy for an individual suffering from glyphosate exposure. Medicine must be a combination of strategies addressing both the quality of the water in which the dolphins swim and individual treatment of the sick dolphin. Let's quickly review what I am proposing as the steps that have led us into this morass of the autoimmune epidemic of our times.

But before discussing treatment, let's briefly recap the origins of autoimmunity, which starts in the gut with the deterioration of both the gut microbiome and the gut lining. Most Americans have deteriorated gut microbiomes because of widespread use of antibiotics in our food system, poor-quality food grown in poor-quality soil, reliance on C-sections and formula feeding, and other factors that either diminish the health and diversity of the microbiome or fail to establish it in the first place. Vaccines also lower the diversity of the microbiome and contain ingredients (see appendix B), such as glyphosate, that make the gut lining more porous. They also shift the immune response to a predominant antibody-producing mode.

Once the gut microbiome is altered and the gut lining becomes porous, large macromolecules that should never have access to the bloodstream begin to show up in the blood. This antigen exposure provokes an antibody response from the person, shifting them even further into a dominant antibody-producing mode. At that point, we have an imbalanced immune system prone to creating excessive inflammatory reactions directed against its own tissues. Once this cross-reactivity starts, the symptoms of dysfunction appear. If the inflammatory attack is directed against the lining of the lungs, we start to see symptoms of asthma. If the inflammatory attack is directed against the joints, we have rheumatoid arthritis.

These excessive inflammatory reactions will often involve not only a heightened antibody response, but also the entire immune system, resulting in cell-mediated tissue destruction. This cell-mediated reaction is the body's attempt to flush out the toxins and antigens that have leaked into our blood, tissues, and cells. These toxins interfere with the ability of the water in our cells to form into healthy cytoplasm, which is the basis of cellular function. A cell with dissolved mercury intercalated into the gel will be a distorted cell with poor function. The body uses its cell-mediated immune function to dissolve the gel, often with fever, as a detoxification response to clear the mercury. The consequence of this cell-mediated activation is also inflammatory damage to the cells involved.

The sequence of events becomes exacerbated and chronic because tissue destruction releases antigens unique to the involved tissue—for example, cartilage antigens in the case of rheumatoid arthritis—into the bloodstream. These antigens provoke further antibody production to neutralize the new antigens in the bloodstream, and the cycle continues.

There is a therapy that could put this situation back into a healthier balance. As a way of introducing it, I am sharing the stories, in their own words, of a few patients who followed the protocol. I have long felt that every patient should talk to others in a similar situation before choosing a course of action. Patients suffering from any particular disease usually know best what works, how long it will take, and what to expect along the way.

These particular patients are adults, but I have given low dose naltrexone (LDN) to children as young as eighteen months, and I have given Restore to very young children as well, often with good results. The important thing is that anyone with an injury or suspected injury from vaccines or an autoimmune or immune system imbalance disorder needs to be seen and monitored by a health practitioner who is well versed in the understanding and treatment of immune-related disorders. This is especially true for very young children, who need not only someone specifically with autoimmune expertise but also someone offering personal, individualized care.

Patient One

I had been suffering for years with a severe and debilitating case of pemphigus. This autoimmune disease targets the skin and membranes in the body. I had large and painful blisters over most of my body—even inside my mouth and throat, as well as very large open sores. My skin looked terrible and was very raw. The slightest pressure on my skin would cause new blisters to erupt. I became unable to walk and I was bedridden and very weak. At times I felt close to death. I didn't want to pursue conventional treatment—it didn't make sense to me to further weaken my immune system—and conventional doctors believe this disease is incurable. I refused to believe that what I had could not be cured.

I am a scientist and I read all I could and researched different treatments, but nothing I tried seemed to produce results. I was treated by two respected "natural" doctors with nutritional treatments and diets but this was a waste of time and I saw no improvement. I came across the work of Dr. Price, which greatly interested me, and this led me to Dr. Cowan. When I first spoke with him, I immediately felt optimistic by the way he was approaching my illness. He started me on the GAPS diet and we tried a few different things to determine what best strengthened my immune system, including low dose naltrexone. I have been taking naltrexone for some time now and feel it has significantly helped in stopping the occurrence of blisters and sores. I am currently taking colostrum in addition to naltrexone and the GAPS diet and I take a few other supplements.

I am now free of pemphigus. I have no blisters anywhere on my body, and my skin and all the open sores have healed. I healed from my head downward and from my head to my knees my skin is now normal. From my knees to my toes it is very nearly normal. It is continuing to improve and I am confident it will soon be equal to my upper body. My energy is excellent. I am exercising and working with a physical therapist and I expect to be walking again. I am very grateful to Dr. Cowan and feel it is truly a miracle when I think about the condition I was in not that long ago with a supposedly incurable autoimmune disease.

Patient Two
It is New Year's Day 2009 and I have recently turned 38. I'm happy because my husband Rick and I are finally in a place in our lives in which we both feel good about beginning to try to

conceive. I want very much to have a child and imagine myself pregnant within the months to come.

We are visiting family up north and that day I go to my cousin's house to try out her new hot tub. We have a lovely visit, but that night I don't sleep a wink. Something in the chemicals in the hot tub seems to have affected me badly and I feel as though I've been drugged. Little do I know that this is a harbinger of difficult times ahead.

Soon after, severe insomnia becomes the norm for me. Often I can sleep from 10 to 12 but then I lie awake until 4 or 5 in the morning, falling back asleep just in time to wake up and get ready for work.

When I do sleep I wake up drenched in sweat. The sheets are soaked. Could this be early perimenopause? That thought terrifies me—I want to have a child so badly. Rather than admit something is wrong I go into denial about it. Not the smartest move, but a fairly typical one for me. When I lie awake at night I experience strong heart palpitations. I think that if someone was looking at me they would surely be able to see my heart beating under my skin.

Other symptoms follow. Muscle and joint pain, intense fatigue during the day, chronic nausea, a sense of restlessness and anxiety. I'm also very thin despite eating as much food as my husband, who weighs 50 pounds more than me. The most common metaphor I use is that I feel as though a motor is revving too high inside of me. It's like the off switch is broken.

I'm feeling completely rotten and maintaining denial requires a fair degree of ingenuity and dedication. In fact I feel so bad that my resourcefulness with this begins to wane (thank goodness!), so I make an appointment with my primary care doctor hoping for some answers. She tells me there is nothing wrong with me. My tests look fine. My hormones are normal. There is no reason she can see for my symptoms or for my apparent inability to get pregnant. I am shocked and confused. Also relieved. Maybe things aren't as bad as I think they are? Thanks for helping rebuild the firewall of denial, Doc! For the better part of the next year I keep trying to tweak my diet, change my exercise routine, and try different herbs, thinking that perhaps I just need some lifestyle adjustments and then I'll feel better and get pregnant. No dice. I feel increasingly despondent as my health deteriorates and as each month passes without being pregnant.

2010. We've been trying to get pregnant for a year. There are days when I'm barely functional I'm so exhausted. (Don't ask me how I think I can be a parent in this condition! Whatever is going on in my body is also affecting my thinking.) One night as I'm lying awake, desperate for sleep but wide awake and buzzing, I begin kicking the wall and sobbing uncontrollably. I feel so afraid, alone, and hopeless. I think I might lose my mind if I don't start sleeping better.

Rick and I make an appointment with a functional medicine practitioner who is also an acupuncturist. She runs the same tests my primary care doctor ran months ago and tells me that I have an autoimmune thyroid condition. I take these tests to my doctor and tell her what I've been told. She looks skeptical. When she looks at my tests she tells me they don't indicate autoimmune thyroid illness. I point out the sky-high thyroid antibodies. She still says they don't mean I have an autoimmune thyroid condition. She is clearly not happy that an acupuncturist thinks they know more than she does. I ask for a referral to the endocrinologist and she begrudgingly writes it up.

The endocrinologist tells me I have Graves' disease. Not only is this an autoimmune hyperthyroid condition, it's one that can kill you. The endocrinologist tells me I can either have my thyroid radioactively ablated or take toxic medication that suppresses the thyroid. These words bounce around the office and I just can't let them land anywhere near me. Everything in me says no, hell, no. She recognizes that neither are good options for someone wanting to get pregnant. I am in shock. I go into the hallway and cry.

In May 2010 my husband tells me to go see Dr. Cowan, who he knows is working with low dose naltrexone. It seems worth a try.

Dr. Cowan tells me that success with LDN and Graves' is variable. He mentions, though, that doctors in Ireland are using it to treat infertility. He suggests that, in addition to taking it, I go on the GAPS diet, which I've done in the past. I begin the diet immediately. I do acupuncture and herbs as well. When the LDN arrives I am eager to begin. Dr. Cowan has suggested that I start at half the dose and take it in the morning since sleep is such a big issue and some people find it interferes with sleep. Full of hope, I take my first half-pill. The next day I feel like a different person. For real.

Within a couple of months of being back on the GAPS diet and taking LDN, my symptoms are entirely gone. The turn-around feels miraculous. For the first two weeks I experienced a headache and wild and wacky dreams. But after two weeks these things settle down. I begin to sleep. The night sweats subside and my energy is returning. I'm no longer struggling with constant pain and nausea. The heart palpitations slow down, but still sometimes occur, although with less and less frequency. My endocrinologist is shocked that I've experienced such a turn-around without conventional treatment. She says she's never seen anything like it. My thyroid levels are exactly where she thinks they ought to be. She is happy though and tells me to continue doing whatever this is that I'm doing. It always strikes me as strange that she doesn't want to know more about it.

In November of 2010 I am thrilled to discover I am pregnant. I will turn 40 in December and I'm really happy that I will be celebrating my birthday feeling healthy and pregnant! Dr. Cowan had suggested that if I got pregnant I might consider going off LDN. I'm scared to do this. I read up on the doctors using it for fertility in Ireland and they say that in the years they have been using it the only difference that they have seen in the babies of women who take LDN during pregnancy is that they seem healthier! With Dr. Cowan's support I continue to take LDN throughout my pregnancy and feel great. My thyroid hormone levels are perfect throughout.

Nine months later I give birth at home to a healthy, robust, 8½-pound baby. I have plenty of milk and go on to breastfeed for three years. Six years later I am still taking LDN and still eating a version of the GAPS diet, which is no longer a diet and is simply how I eat. I am symptom-free (although I can make symptoms start to return by eating a lot of grains or sweets). I give thanks all the time for the wonderful health I enjoy and the healthy child who I love.

The Therapy

I. The Cowan Autoimmune Diet or GAPS Diet

The preceding two patients followed a strict GAPS protocol as an important component in healing from their autoimmune disease. The Cowan Autoimmune Diet outlined in chapter 12 is a variant of the standard GAPS diet. Either one is fundamentally an attempt to use food to address the imbalances in the microbiome and gut lining. Variations have been around since the mid-1940s as strategies for healing disorders of the gastrointestinal tract.

The GAPS diet involves cells lining the intestines that produce enzymes called disaccharidases and whose function is to digest disaccharides, otherwise known as starches. When a person has a disordered microbiome, the villi—the tiny hairlike protrusions that line the intestines—become blunted. This blunting compromises the villi's ability to synthesize disaccharidases, resulting in an inability to break down and therefore digest starches.

If someone continues to eat these disaccharide-containing foods—grains, beans, and some other starchy foods such as potatoes—these incompletely digested foods will remain in the gastrointestinal tract, becoming food for yeast and other pathogens that normally reside in smaller numbers within the intestinal lumen. This further weakens the microbiome, leading to further erosion of the gut wall, deterioration of the villi, and even less ability to synthesize disaccharidases and digest starches.

This vicious cycle can only be broken by complete elimination of disaccharides from the diet, the avoidance of toxins, such as glyphosate, that compromise gut function, and a dietary program designed to restore a healthy, diverse microbiome.

In the Cowan Autoimmune Diet, all disaccharides are eliminated for the first six months, sometimes longer if the healing needs more time. At the same time, the gut flora is nourished by the consumption of healthy fats, a wide diversity of vegetables, including a daily serving of leeks, and daily consumption of lacto-fermented foods from both vegetable (e.g., sauerkraut) and animal (e.g., 24-hour yogurt and kefir) sources. There are many good resources for learning how to make lacto-fermented foods, including *Wild Fermentation* by Sandor Katz, *Gut and Psychology Syndrome* by Natasha Campbell-McBride, and *Nourishing Traditions* by Sally Fallon Morell and Mary G. Enig.

Gut-lining health is supported mainly by the daily inclusion of gelatin-rich bone broth. Gelatin is a rich source of the amino acids that are used as fuel by the intestinal cells and is the traditional food most associated with the restoration of the gut. Chicken broth is the traditional remedy for an inflamed gut (i.e., gastroenteritis). Any source of gelatin-rich broth can be used, as long as it is sourced from organic-pastured bones, because commercial animal products can be a hidden source of glyphosate.

Building your diet around healthy fats, including grass-fed butter, ghee, pastured lard, coconut oil, and organic raw olive oil; grass-fed or pastured eggs or meat; wild-caught fish; a large diversity of vegetables; and minimal amounts of fresh fruit, seeds, and nuts is the essence of the Cowan Autoimmune Diet. Combine these with restriction of disaccharide-containing foods for six months and a patient is well on her way to restoring her gut microbiome and better health.

II. Low Dose Naltrexone

I rarely prescribe pharmaceutical drugs. The only exception is a remarkable medicine called low dose naltrexone (LDN), which

I have been prescribing for two decades. The beneficial effects I've seen from LDN are unparalleled by any other therapy or approach I know.

Naltrexone was first synthesized in the 1960s, following the search for an antidote to heroin overdose among servicemen and servicewomen returning to the United States from Vietnam. Naltrexone is an opiate receptor antagonist, meaning that it prevents the activity of opiates by blocking the opioid receptors, located primarily in the brain, spinal cord, and digestive tract. Naltrexone has a low "agonist" effect; that is, it effectively blocks the action of the opiate without producing any opiate effect of its own, unlike, for example, methadone. Over time, naltrexone, which is commonly sold under the trade name Narcan, became the drug of choice to reverse heroin overdose. This has been a great success, saving countless lives, and continues to be used in this capacity to this day.

In the 1970s and 1980s, clinicians and researchers began to explore naltrexone not only in cases of acute overdoses but also in the treatment of opiate (and alcohol) addiction, typically with a dosage of 50 milligrams a day, which largely blocks the psychoactive effect (i.e., the high) of the opiate. At first, this seemed like an exciting and promising strategy, but by and large it ultimately failed in the treatment of addiction because addicts overwhelmingly reported feeling so lousy that they didn't want to take it.

This would have been the end of naltrexone, except as a short-acting antidote to opiate overdose, if not for some astute clinicians and researchers who began wondering why naltrexone made addicts feel so uniformly lousy. This line of questioning led to the discovery and understanding of endorphins, which are essentially endogenous (read: produced internally) opiates. Heroin and the other opiates don't work because we're born with opiate receptors; they work because we're born with endorphin receptors that opiates co-opt. Endorphin receptors are some of the most ubiquitous receptors in the human body, particularly in nervous system and immune system cells, and endorphins are essential to our nervous system, our immune system, and our emotional lives. When you block their effect by blocking receptors—as you can with a 50-milligram-a-day dose of naltrexone—you produce dysfunction of the nervous system, the immune system, and emotional life.

Again, this might have been the end of naltrexone as a medicine but for an astute New York City physician named Bernard Bihari, who noticed that many of his severely immune-compromised patients, including those suffering from AIDS and lymphoma, were also heroin or opiate addicts. He wondered whether the replacement of one's own endorphins with exogenously sourced opiates, usually heroin, was the source of their immune dysfunction. He began searching for a way to boost endorphin levels in his patients suffering from diseases related to immune dysfunction.

After years of experimentation, Bihari discovered that if he gave a very small dose of naltrexone, particularly right before going to bed, his patients experienced significant improvement in immune function and general well-being. *The LDN Book*, by Linda Elsegood, details research into the use of low dose naltrexone to increase endorphin levels in the blood, improving immune function, lowering antibody levels, and even putting a variety of autoimmune diseases into remission.

LDN is a pharmaceutical trick, but a highly effective one. As is the case with a high dose of naltrexone, LDN blocks opiate/endorphin receptors. The difference is that with a very small dose, the naltrexone block lasts only a few hours and occurs while a patient is sleeping. The body tries to overcome this receptor blockade by increasing production of endogenous opiates—that is, endorphins. When the patient wakes up, it's with more endorphins in the blood, resulting in more energy and a greater sense of well-being—just as she might experience from intense running, acupuncture, or chocolate.

More to our point, not only does she feel better, she also has a significant, often dramatic, and often almost immediate improvement and normalization in immune function. Specifically, LDN seems to lower antibody levels, calming the humoral immune response while stimulating cell-mediated reactivity. This is exactly what we want to achieve in any therapy for autoimmune disease. As a result of this cell-mediated activity, a person can detoxify more efficiently, lowering the antibody levels associated with a chronic inflammatory response that characterizes autoimmune disease.

Over the past decade I have treated hundreds of patients with the combination of diet and LDN. Many of these patients have experienced full remission from a wide range of autoimmune diseases. The most common forms of autoimmune diseases I have treated in this way are Crohn's disease, ulcerative colitis, psoriasis, Hashimoto's thyroiditis, asthma, eczema, and multiple sclerosis. I have used LDN in patients from eighteen-month-olds—including a baby suffering from juvenile rheumatoid arthritis who experienced complete remission in three months and hasn't relapsed in seven years—to octogenarians. During this time, I have seen no significant side effects or complications from LDN, including no elevations in liver enzymes and no rashes, with the exception of occasional difficulty sleeping that can usually be resolved by lowering the dose.

The rule of thumb about dosing is the lower the better. The "standard" dose is 4.5 milligrams before bed, but I often start with 1.5 milligrams or even less, particularly with children. If there is a positive response, I maintain that dose for at least a year. If there is no response after a month, I generally increase the dose to 3 milligrams for a month and then assess the response. If there is still no response by the beginning of the third month, I increase the dose to 4.5 milligrams and continue that dose for six months. About 20 percent of my patients will see no appreciable improvement in six months with a combination of diet therapy and LDN. Usually these are patients who have been on long-term prednisone therapy or other immune-suppressive drugs. For them, I will continue for as long as a year before concluding that this therapy is not helpful for them.

For the 80 percent who do respond, they often describe it as life changing. For them, I typically continue the LDN for at least three years, and certainly until they have been off all conventional medicines for at least one year. At that point, it can make sense to stop the LDN and assess the patient's response. Some of my patients have been on LDN for over a decade with continued effectiveness and complete absence of side effects or toxicity. (Patients are sometimes erroneously told by doctors that it will hurt their liver.)

Some patients benefit from occasional two-week breaks, but this is rarely necessary. I am convinced from my study of the relevant research on LDN and my personal experience that every patient suffering from any autoimmune disease, including autism, lupus, Hashimoto's thyroiditis, and rheumatoid arthritis, should at some point try a combination of the Cowan Autoimmune Diet and LDN, certainly before moving on to toxic conventional treatments.

The Cowan Autoimmune Diet and LDN form the foundation of my treatment for all autoimmune diseases. This, along with complete avoidance of vaccines, acetaminophen, and anti-inflammatory drugs. In addition, patients should spend plenty of time in nature—particularly in bare feet, such as walking on the beach—and sunshine. This is often all someone needs to experience a tremendous change in the course of their condition. That said, there are also other natural medicines and interventions that I use and will discuss, because they can also have an impact on various conditions.

III. Restore

Developed by Dr. Zach Bush and his team of researchers in Virginia, Restore is a soil-derived supplement that can decrease zonulin levels, reducing leakage through the gut wall. Zonulin, discovered and described in 2000, is a protein that modulates permeability through the gut wall, ideally preventing the absorption of antigens and toxins.[2] Glyphosate and some components of vaccines will increase zonulin concentrations in the gut, essentially "telling" pores in the gut wall to open. As a result of this excessive signal for the gut wall to open, the intestinal lining becomes overly porous, initiating autoimmune dysfunction.

Restore seems to work by lowering zonulin concentrations and sealing the gut wall. I have seen success with it, particularly in pediatric patients suffering from eczema and asthma, typically associated with food allergies and vaccine exposure. In the space of a month, during which a patient completely avoids glyphosate-containing foods—at least as much as is possible these days—and takes ½ to 1 teaspoon of Restore three times a day a half hour before each meal, I have seen the eczema and asthma clear up completely. Restore works on one of the fundamental pathologies of autoimmune disease—leaky gut—and is worth considering for anyone suffering from any kind of autoimmune disease.

IV. Colostrum

At its best, natural medicine attempts to re-create the body's own healing strategies. If the body is using pus to expel a splinter, an appropriate therapy is to simply help the body by removing the splinter. The body's appreciation can be seen in the disappearance of the pus, often within hours. Once we've eliminated the body's need to use heroic means—pus, fever, and other immune activation—to rid itself of the splinter, the situation resolves itself quietly and the big guns are no longer needed.

With autoimmune diseases, the body's need is to restore a healthy gut ecosystem. In a healthy scenario, an individual's microbiome is established as he passes through his mother's birth canal. With this the baby swallows his mother's vaginal secretion, thereby "seeding" his own microbiome and the foundation of his immune system.

Then something amazing and surprising happens: For the next two or three days the baby eats colostrum, a nonnutritive food, at a moment when it seems like nourishment would be urgently needed. And yet, this first milk is crucial for the survival of virtually all mammals. What's happening? The colostrum is primarily providing nutrients and growth factors for the establishing microbial community. That is, before a mammalian baby nourishes himself, he must establish and nourish his microbiome. This is incredible if you think about it: We're feeding our bacteria before we're feeding ourselves. And the reason is that these bacteria are crucial to our survival—they will form the basis of a growing immune system. Once the microbes have been happily sated—or are at least on their way to being solidly established, the breast milk has come in and the baby will find nourishment within it. Many mammals, including pigs, horses, cats, and dogs, won't survive if they are deprived of colostrum.[3] Human babies survive, but their gut flora may be compromised for life.

A person with disturbed gut flora can benefit from a daily serving of fresh (preferably) or powdered colostrum—or may even embark on a two- to three-day colostrum fast to simulate the immediate perinatal period in which the microbiome and foundation of the immune system are established. It's difficult for most people to find a source of fresh colostrum, but I provide some sources for powdered colostrum, which is a reasonable substitute, in recommended resources. The dose is generally one teaspoon two to three times a day for children up to the age of nine and one tablespoon two to three times a day for adults and children over the age of nine.

V. Organ Preparations

One of the factors that perpetuates the autoimmune cycle is the inflammatory destruction of affected tissue, such as the thyroid in Hashimoto's thyroiditis or the cartilage in rheumatoid arthritis, that causes nuclear material (including DNA) of the destroyed tissue to spill into the blood. This causes the body to produce antibodies against this nuclear material, which then goes on to create more inflammation against that tissue. And the vicious cycle continues.

One way to break this vicious cycle is to use a kind of decoy. Many antibodies are produced in lymph tissues surrounding the gut, called Peyer's patches, so that if you eat tissue from an animal that is the same kind of tissue your antibodies are targeting, it is possible that your Peyer's patches will make antibodies that attack the orally ingested tissue and leave your own organ alone. This technique is called oral tolerance therapy.

For example, in Hashimoto's thyroiditis or Graves' disease the targeted tissue is the thyroid gland, so if a patient eats thyroid extract from a cow, whose cells and DNA are very similar, some of the attack will be directed against the extract instead of the patient's thyroid gland. This gives the patient's thyroid a chance to heal and, for many patients, has proven to be an invaluable aid in restoring function to a stressed gland. I generally use grass-fed organ preparations from a California-based supplement company called Allergy Research. These organ preparations are best taken without food, between meals, and in an amount of anywhere from one to four capsules two to three times a day.

The preceding program is my basic autoimmune protocol. At times, I will add other specific herbs or nutrients or even foods for a particular patient on a case-by-case basis. But for more than 90 percent of my patients—men, women, and children—the simple strategy outlined herein is sufficient for significant improvement in health and in the course of an autoimmune condition.

CHAPTER TWELVE

The Cowan Autoimmune Diet

The Cowan Autoimmune Diet is based on the etiology of autoimmune disease as I describe it in this book. For example, one of the first steps in the progression of any autoimmune disease is disturbance in the gut microbiome; this can be addressed through a proper diet. Another factor is deterioration of the intestinal villi; this can also be addressed through a proper diet. The principles in the Cowan Autoimmune Diet are by no means unique; they can be found in the GAPS diet, the Autoimmune Paleo Diet, and the Wahls Protocol. These are all wonderful dietary approaches and I have used each of them successfully in my many years of treating people with autoimmune diseases.

I have a slightly different take than these other approaches, which I've developed in my role not only as a physician treating patients with autoimmune diseases but also as a gardener. In fact, my interest in gardening led me directly to found, along with my family, our vegetable business, Dr. Cowan's Garden. Caring for plants and the soil in which plants are grown has done more to educate me about food and healing than all the reading and studying I have ever done. It's one thing to speculate and think about health; it's quite a different experience to watch one's garden suffer because of compacted garden beds.

The other perspective I bring comes from my emphasis on water. Water molecules make up more than 99.9 percent of the molecules in our bodies. And the state of our health is in many ways a result of how well we are able to structure this water in our cells and tissues. Human beings are complex and often it is not easy to see directly the effects of any particular intervention. Plants are complex as well, but the effects of various practices, such as using compost or structuring the water you use to irrigate your plants, are easier to see. Experiences in my years of gardening have led me to formulate some of the principles in this diet.

Finally, while the thrust of this book is on the understanding and treatment of autoimmune diseases, and this diet is considered a part of that therapy, we must never lose sight of the importance of finding joy in our lives. Food is an integral part, in every culture and society, in the attainment of this joy. The sensual quality of food, including not just its taste, but its aroma and appearance, is an essential part of this diet and an essential part of any true healing. Our quest should be for a life of abundance, joy, and meaning. There is no greater venue for executing this quest than in our relationship with food. With that introduction, here are the principles of the Cowan Autoimmune Diet.

Food Quality

In some ways, in a list of the top ten dietary principles, attention to food quality should be numbers one through nine. As there is such an intimate connection between pesticide or herbicide use and diseases, including polio and autism, it is imperative for anyone suffering from any autoimmune disease, or any disease of any kind, to pay strict attention to the quality of food they're eating. By "quality," I refer not only to the care of soil and pastures that forms the foundation of healthy food, but also to more subtle aspects, such as the correct time to harvest vegetables and the proper way to store and process the foods we eat.

I know many people don't have access to the quality of food I'm suggesting, but my hope in laying out these guidelines is that our society, especially the agricultural community, eventually incorporates these principles into common practice. I would like to see us stop considering food a commodity and instead develop a more creative economic system for the production of the healthiest food, making it freely available to anyone who wants it. We're a long way off from this, but it's not too early to sound the call for change.

When I talk about quality I don't only mean the vitamin, mineral, or nutrient content of food. My longtime gardening experience has convinced me that different practices in fertilizing, composting, and irrigation can lead to very different outcomes in terms of flavor. I garden for flavor and trust that nutrient content will follow; our sense of flavor tells us a great deal about nutrient content and density. As time goes on, if you make a commitment to eating only real foods, ones that are properly grown, your sense of taste and smell will deepen and your ability to sense food quality will grow. This will directly improve your health. A commitment to food quality needs to be a total commitment—meaning the complete abandonment of inferior-quality foods. Here are the "rules":

a. The best food is properly foraged or caught wild. This means the forager or hunter needs to be aware of sustainable foraging practices and must avoid contaminated land and water. The hunter needs to be aware of how to humanely kill and dress his prey. The next-best quality will come from pastured animals, followed by food grown on biodynamic farms or gardens or on small-scale permaculture farms. Following that is food produced by small-scale family farms or gardens or food grown in your own organic homestead or garden. The final acceptable source is food grown on large-scale certified organic farms. For help finding these types of foods, the Weston A. Price Foundation shopping guide can be invaluable (see recommended resources).

b. Processing should either be not at all or by traditional techniques that have stood the test of time. Foods that undergo no processing include fresh salad or cucumbers right from the garden or farmer's market. Examples of traditional processing techniques, which in many cases enhance the quality of the food, include traditional lacto-fermentation; making butter or fermented dairy products (e.g., kefir, yogurt) from pastured, 100 percent grass-fed whole milk; or the production of traditionally cured meat products such as bacon or prosciutto. Other quality-enhancing processing techniques include making sourdough bread from freshly ground heirloom grains, soaking or sprouting of seeds and nuts, and making lacto-fermented drinks from excess garden produce. These and many more techniques for enhancing food quality can be found in the book *Nourishing Traditions*, by Sally Fallon Morell and Mary G. Enig.

c. Finally, and especially relevant to those who have their own gardens, leaf and fruit vegetables such as kale, lettuce, zucchini, and peppers should be harvested as early in the morning as possible, whereas root vegetables such as carrots, beets, parsnips, and horseradish are best harvested in the evening. While this may seem like a small point, the energy of the plant is most concentrated in the leaves early in the morning, enhancing the flavor and allowing them to be stored longer in the refrigerator. On the other hand, through the day the energy and nutrient flow of the plant drops down into the roots, so root vegetables will store and retain their freshness longer when harvested in the evening.

Macronutrient Content

Dietary macronutrient content refers to the proportion of fats, proteins, and carbohydrates. The optimal relationship of macronutrients in our diet can be loosely described as liberal good fats, modest protein, and low carbohydrate. While I hesitate to give numbers, the best guide is that each meal should contain a sufficient amount of fats. The four main fats to use are grass-fed butter, grass-fed ghee, coconut oil, and olive oil. Other fats and oils that can be included (provided they are the best quality) include lard from pastured pigs, beef tallow, and duck fat. With other plant oils, we run into the problem of extraction and production of most seed and flower oils; most seeds and flowers typically need high-temperature grinding in order to extract the oils. This high-heat process harms the oils and decreases the nutrient content. The only acceptable quality source I know for true low-heat oil extraction, followed by the preservation of the oil in Miron jars, is a company called Andreas Seed Oils (see recommended resources).

Protein generally comes from a modest serving at each meal of animal products, which can include fish, meat, eggs, whole-milk raw cheeses, or organ meats. By "modest," I mean about the size of a deck of cards; more than that is unnecessary and can create an undue burden on the kidneys. In addition to this portion of protein at each meal, soup or bone broth from any quality animal source should also be included. Everyone should eat at least one cup of gelatin-containing broth each day; those with an autoimmune disease should eat one cup up to three times a day. The gelatin proteins in bone broth are key for healing and sealing the gut and are therefore at the core of my autoimmune treatment program. All broth should come from the bones of 100 percent grass-fed, pastured animals in order to avoid contamination from chemicals such as glyphosate that are found in all commercial animal feed. There are almost no exceptions to this.

Finally, carbohydrate content should be low. This is the only time I give people a specific number: generally between 45 and 75 grams of net carbohydrates per day. There are many good books, particularly those that advocate very low carbohydrate or ketogenic diets, that can guide you in how to count carbohydrate grams in your diet. Fats are a more efficient fuel for our bodies than carbohydrates are, and our true need for dietary carbohydrates is small. As advocated for in the GAPS diet, most people with an active autoimmune disease should go six months without any disaccharides, which means the elimination of all grains and beans. In my autoimmune diet, I, too, counsel patients to start with a six-month elimination of grains, beans, and nonfermented milk products. This allows the opportunity for significant gut microbiome restoration. Carbohydrate consumption during this time comes from vegetables such as carrots, beets, or parsnips, and a small amount of fruit. These carbohydrates, in addition to the meats and fats and green vegetables, provide you with all the nutrients, fiber, and vitamins that you need.

Lacto-Fermented Foods

The microorganisms that make up healthy gut flora are originally introduced into our GI tract during passage through the birth canal. This is followed by two or three days of colostrum from our mothers, which contains growth factors that help these microbes grow and flourish in our GI tract. Then, through skin contact, eating microbes in food, and contact with soil and the rest of the natural world, we gradually establish a diverse, healthy microbiome throughout our lives. When signs of trouble such as autoimmune symptoms emerge, we must redouble our efforts to introduce these beneficial microbes into our GI tract. We can play in soil, gardens, and compost, particularly with our bare hands, and eat an abundant supply of as great a diversity of microbes as possible. Our adaptation to place is crucial.

When I say "adaptation to place," I mean that throughout the history of humankind, people connected with and adapted to their homeland through interaction with unique soil and food. They worked the soil and fermented their own produce in their homes and villages. Doing so literally connects us to the life of the place we live and is one of the foundations of health. We can re-create this to a certain extent by bringing the art of fermentation back into our homes. Many wonderful books have been written about how to ferment foods, but none are better than *The Art of Fermentation*, by Sandor Katz. Daily consumption of as wide a variety of lacto-fermented foods, preferably home or locally made, is key in the restoration of health. Start with fermented vegetables such as sauerkraut, beet kvass, and kimchi, and then move to homemade cultured dairy products, fruits, and other beverages. For those with the inclination, even the traditional fermentation of meat and other animal products will increase the diversity in your diet and microbial consumption. Eat at least a small amount of fermented vegetables or drinks with each meal and, depending on your tolerance, increase consumption of traditional lacto-fermented foods to about 10 percent of your daily diet. Over time, just this change is an effective step in the restoration of a healthy, diverse microbiome.

Diversity

Exposure to as wide a variety of foods as possible is the key to ensuring that you will consume all the vitamins, minerals, phytonutrients, and other disease-prevention agents you need that the plant and animal world makes available to us. I have been trying to incorporate this principle in my life for decades, to the point of counting precisely how many different plants I eat in a month. The key to this is to eat seasonally, grow your own garden, include perennials, and use herbs and spices liberally in cooking. Everyone should spend a month keeping track of their personal diversity consumption; aim for between twelve and fifteen different plants each day and between sixty and eighty each month. Eat widely from all the healthy animal products available in your area. Connect with a hunter in your area to have access to otherwise unavailable wild game and other hard-to-obtain animal products. Be creative and learn to use wild foods in flavorful dishes. In so doing you reaffirm your connection to the world of nature around you.

Water

I put a lot of emphasis on the quality of water in our cells, tissues, and bodily fluids such as blood, lymph, and cerebrospinal fluid. The quality of the water in our bodies is related to the quality of water we consume in our food and drinks. The best water is highly mineralized, highly structured at a temperature of around 4° Celsius, which is generally only attainable from glacier runoff in the few remaining pristine places on earth. So, knowing that the perfect solution to water consumption doesn't exist, we need to try and obtain the best possible water for our bodies.

When you choose a water source, the water should contain as few contaminants as possible. This includes everything from the fluoride and chlorine/chloramines put in most municipal water supplies, to such things as pharmaceutical drugs and agricultural chemicals. Besides getting the "stuff" out of the water, healthy water should be in motion, particularly in a spiral motion. Water in a spiral motion, as it often exists in nature, is energized and structured. In plant experiments, it's been shown that watering plants with structured, vortexed water increases the vigor and health of the plants. I have frequently been impressed when observing positive health effects in my patients who commit to consuming only structured water.

The best option I know of for obtaining the best-quality water for home consumption is to start with your tap water. Add one teaspoon of Adya Clarity to a gallon of tap water and let this sit for at least twenty-four hours. The Adya Clarity contains a kind of "clay" that binds to most contaminants in the water, including chlorine, fluoride, and most pharmaceutical drugs. You will see a yellow precipitate as the bound contaminants fall out of solution. Strain the precipitate using a normal carbon-based filter and then run this water through a vortex/remineralization machine such as the Tribest Duet Water Revitalizer. This structures and adds minerals back into the water. Then put the water into either Miron bottles or Flaska water bottles and keep them in the refrigerator.

Trust Your Instincts

The final principle of the Cowan Autoimmune Diet is for you to use yourself as the most important feedback device in determining which foods work best for you. Understanding the effects foods have on you is a skill that improves with practice and commitment. The commitment here is to pay attention and honor your instincts. If you have any sense that a certain food doesn't agree with you, skip it for at least a week, then try it again and pay close attention to how you feel after eating it. Gradually your instincts will sharpen and become clearer, but only if you make an absolute commitment to pay attention and honor your inner voice that informs how you react and feel related to your food intake. Sharpening of instincts happens to everyone who makes an absolute commitment to eating real foods; with this commitment you will be well on your way to having a unique diet, designed for you, by you, that works for you. Commitment is the holy grail of dietary therapy.

To summarize, these six dietary principles should get you off to a good start in organizing your autoimmune diet. For the first six months omit all grains, beans, and noncultured dairy products, which can then slowly be reintroduced. Be creative in the procurement, processing, and final preparation of your foods. Enjoy your meals, make mealtime a family and connection time, and consult the various books on traditional foods that I recommend for further ideas on the organization of your daily diet.

Sample Daily Menus: First Six Months

Breakfast

The simplest and most nutritious breakfast for those on the Cowan Autoimmune Diet is freshly made soup with 6–10 sautéed vegetables in any of the allowed fats with added bone broth. Add salt or powdered sea vegetables to taste. Then add a big dollop of sauerkraut or any other fermented vegetables on top. In addition, 2 eggs cooked in any way you like. To vary this basic breakfast, just change the vegetables in the soup, or change the eggs to a small amount of naturally made meat, fish, or sausage. Finish your breakfast with 2–4 ounces of homemade beet kvass.

Lunch

For many, this can be a light meal, something like a large snack. Again, the components are simple. Start with a deck-of-cards-sized animal food, such as raw milk cheese (if you tolerate dairy products), fish, meat, or some other protein. Always consume protein with adequate fats—meaning only full-fat dairy products and more fatty cuts of meat and fish. Then add lots of vegetables—steamed, sautéed, raw (if you tolerate raw vegetables), fermented, and so forth. Add a sauce or dressing that contains some fat to the vegetables, as this will help you absorb the nutrients in them. This can include adding avocados, a wonderful source of fats, or a sauce or dressing made with olive oil or cultured cream. Use herbs and spices liberally on your food and vary the vegetables seasonally and to taste. Finally, the various berries and high-phytonutrient fruits such as pome-granates or persimmons, when in season, are a good source of nutrient-rich carbohydrates.

Dinner

Dinner on the Cowan Autoimmune Diet is a hybrid of breakfast and lunch. What works best for most people is to start the meal with a cup of stew or soup made with a base of bone broth and various vegetables. To this, add a deck-of-cards-sized protein, vegetables cooked and fermented in a variety of ways, and a dessert of a small amount of berries or seasonal fruit with a small amount of cultured cream.

After the First Six Months

After the first six months, once significant health restoration has occurred, and being careful to observe any negative reactions, you can add a small amount of soaked or sprouted grains and beans. At first, continue to omit gluten-containing grains, but over time they may also be reintroduced into your diet. Aim for an inclusive diet, as long as it is grounded in food quality. Start with simple rice, sprouted quinoa, and soaked lentils. Add these foods to each meal in small quantities and gradually increase your repertoire to include heirloom and even perennial grains daily. Slowly build up to a full *Nourishing Traditions*–type of diet, characterized by flavor, nutrient density, diversity, and ecological restoration, and enjoy the process as you go.

Conclusion

uthor and philosopher Ivan Illich remarked that two of the worst things one person can do to another person—especially a child—is convince him that in order to learn he must be taught (read: schooled) and that in order to heal he must be doctored.

We know, however, that most children will easily learn their native language without ever being explicitly taught. If an adult wants to be involved, all she needs to do is engage with a child in the usual way humans interact, and the child will naturally learn to speak. Given the chance, most human beings *love* to learn. Each person does so in a slightly different way, with a focus on different things and with different interests. The most effective way to disengage a child from learning is to force her to learn what you, the adult, think is good for her, in the rhythm and style that you think is best. Healthy children resist and rebel against this abrogation of their freedom and autonomy; less healthy children submit and become schooled.

Not long ago, my wife Lynda and I went on a vacation for a week at a lakeside cottage in New Hampshire with two of our grandchildren, Ben and Sam, ages five and four. At the beginning of the week, neither boy knew how to swim. The lake was shallow, but the boys were hesitant and clung to their inflatable rafts. Ignoring my best instincts, I figured that if they learned to swim, our vacation would be a lot more fun. So I tried to teach them. They ignored me, of course, and began complaining about many and various things.

I mustered the sense to back off and let them be. Within two days, both boys were effective dog-paddlers and could swim underwater for ten feet. While I sat peacefully on the beach, they began diving off their little rafts, showing me their newest exploits.

Likewise, most of us have experienced a small cut or infection that easily healed without medicine or intervention. A human being is fundamentally a self-healing system. Infections are the body's way of detoxifying, and fever is the most effective prevention and treatment strategy ever devised. You don't have to teach a child how to get a fever; it comes naturally, as part of the original design.

Our job as parents, doctors, and caretakers for children is mostly to observe and, only when needed, help guide a process to its healthy conclusion. But mostly we don't. We intervene. We manage. We attempt to control. Doing something, anything, temporarily assuages our fears (and creates massive industries in the process). The result, however, is much like what Ivan Illich predicted: a medicalized society that must devote huge resources to dealing with sick people; as the amount of medicine in our world increases, so, too, does the amount of sickness. Beyond a certain basic level of care, use of more medicine not only undermines an individual's freedom and autonomy, but also degrades a society's health.

Recently, a new patient came to me with a rheumatological complaint. She said her primary care physician referred her to a rheumatologist, but that the first new patient appointment was more than six months away. The rheumatology business must be booming if the supply of new patients with debilitating joint disease so drastically outstrips the number of doctors who are available to treat it.

The cost of medical care in most of the developed world is threatening to bankrupt us. The strategy we're using to prevent disease is not working. It should be *rare* for someone to need doctoring. It should be *unusual* for someone to be so chronically debilitated that they need to consume pharmaceuticals daily in order to be able to function. It should be *uncommon* for someone to have an organ removed from her body in order that she might live and function in the world. These things are not only *not* rare; our economy depends on them. What if there were suddenly no wars, no sick people, and children happily learned on their own? The entire US economy would collapse into a heap of rubble. Once a society finds itself financially dependent on war, sickness, imprisonment, and enforced schooling, it must be understood that the solution to these problems can't be more of the same.

This book is not an in-depth investigation of the illnesses we vaccinate against, a review of studies done to date on vaccine safety or toxicity, or an exploration of all current research on the immunology of vaccines. All of these are important topics; I've included documentaries and books that address them in the recommended resources. Instead, in this book I look more broadly at the connection between vaccines and the nature of autoimmune diseases and, I hope, add another layer to the debate. I explore the consequences—intended and unintended—of subjecting a population to the huge number of vaccines that the CDC currently recommends and that schools and other institutions currently require.

My conclusion, as Illich predicted, is that when we charge forward into the unknown with the idea that we can eradicate disease from human life, the result will be more suffering, more misery, more poverty. Illness, including childhood illness, is a part of the human condition. Illness is the soil in which the development of empathy, compassion, and robust health emerges. Children who go through the fires of childhood illnesses emerge with confidence in their innate ability to heal, which leads to confidence in their ability to be autonomous, self-directed individuals. Children who are prevented from overcoming diseases become increasingly susceptible to greater maladies later in life. And, tragically, they are prevented from undertaking the sacred quest of overcoming the adversity of sickness as they grow into self-confident mature human beings.

We have traded a temporary reduction in (in many cases) innocuous childhood illnesses for a lifetime of toxicity, chronic disease, clouding of the spiritual world, and loss of self-confidence in our ability to heal without intervention.

With vaccination, whether due to greed, corruption, difference of opinion, or scientific debate, we have taken a dramatically wrong turn. If we don't engage in an immediate course correction—a reevaluation not only of our vaccine policies but of the entire field of pediatrics—our society will not be able to withstand the growing burden of sick and disabled citizens.

When scientists predict that, in twenty years, half of all American children will suffer from one or more chronic diseases, it is past time to take stock of who we are, how we live, and what kind of world we want. My hope is that this book helps in this reevaluation and gently nudges more of us toward a way of life aligned with the development of free, autonomous, and spiritually aware human beings.

As a family doctor in New Hampshire I often had little or no contact with children while they were sick, particularly in cases of chicken pox, and only heard about their illness after the fact when I would run into a parent at the playground or a special event. Whooping cough cases were more dramatic and painful, and so I would sometimes treat children who had been suffering for a long time, including my son Joe, who contracted it at eight weeks old and was sick for four months.

With rare exceptions, I never prescribed antibiotics to the children I saw. I generally treated patients with the *Nourishing Traditions* diet,[1] one-half to one teaspoon per day of cod liver oil, liposomal vitamin C hourly in the acute phases, tapering to three to four times per day when the illness receded, and the appropriate homeopathic and/or anthroposophical medicines for each illness. I was fortunate that none of my pediatric patients died or experienced irreparable damage following a childhood illness; both of these outcomes are always possible, and I'm grateful not to have encountered them.

My experience is an extremely small sample of what can happen when children become ill. Life is always a gamble: Bad things can happen. Children can die. They can have adverse outcomes. Nobody wants this. I certainly don't. I don't know anyone who does.

Which is why I'm also grateful to have vaccinated so few children. To vaccinate a child and then witness them die is not something I could ever live with. Children do die from vaccines; the only debate is over how often it happens.[2] Nor could I live with watching a child embark on a potentially lifelong struggle with an autoimmune disease or autism following the administration of a vaccine. The medical establishment and mainstream media continue to deny this outcome, but research continues, evidence is mounting, and many parents have many stories that call into question a stance from the CDC and AAP that relies solely on the brandishing of medical credentials and authority.

I continue to hope for and invite an honest, open, and courteous discussion on this issue, which I believe is the human rights issue of our time.

APPENDIX A

Don't the Scientific Studies Prove That There Is No Causal Connection between Autism and Vaccines?

I hear all the time that numerous studies have shown that vaccines are safe and effective, that this is settled science, that vaccines have been proven not to cause health problems. Most of the time the people who tell me this, including pediatricians, cannot point to a single study that actually proves any such thing. So let's look at two of the most-cited studies by the AAP and the CDC that claim to "prove" that vaccines are safe. For my review of these studies I am indebted to the authors of the website *Vaccine Papers* (vaccinepapers.org), which is a key reference for anyone who is interested in the science behind vaccines. If you or your doctor want to truly understand the scientific literature on vaccines, a thorough reading of the contents of this website is imperative.

The first study is referred to as the "Smith et al. study" and was published in *Pediatrics* in 2010 under the title "On-time Vaccine Receipt in the First Year Does Not Adversely Affect Neuropsychological Outcomes." The conclusion of the study reads: "This study provides the strongest clinical outcomes evidence to date that on-time receipt of vaccines during infancy has no adverse effect on neurodevelopmental outcomes 7 to 10 years later. These results offer reassuring information that physicians and public health officials may use to communicate with parents who are concerned that children receive too many vaccines too soon."[1]

Let's look at the findings. The stated purpose of the study was to look at children who receive their vaccines in a "timely" manner compared to those who receive them in an "untimely" manner. This is a reasonable objective because if one group of children follows the CDC schedule and the other group doesn't, we should be able to ascertain differences in outcome. The study looked at children vaccinated between 1993 and 1997 who were then followed until they were approximately 10 years old. They were assessed between the ages of 7 and 10 to see if they showed any neuropsychological differences, including attention-deficit/hyperactivity disorder, autism, tics, and so forth. So far the research sounds good, but then come the details. The definition of a child with "untimely" vaccines includes having the full CDC schedule of shots but being more than thirty days late on one or more of the suggested vaccines. This means that if a child followed the usual CDC vaccine schedule except for getting one vaccine thirty days late for any reason, they were put in the "untimely" group. Because of this methodology, after the first year the "timely" group had an average of 11.8 vaccines and the "untimely" group had an average of 10.1 vaccines. After the first seven months, the "timely" group had 11.1 shots and the "untimely" group had 8 shots.

A study that purports to show that vaccines are safe and don't cause or correlate with neurodevelopment issues—currently at epidemic levels in our children—is defining children who receive an average of 10.1 of shots in the first year as less vaccinated, or not vaccinated in a "timely" manner. In some interpretations, the "untimely" group is referred to as "unvaccinated." Of course, this small difference between the "timely" and the "untimely" group would naturally be unlikely to show any significant issues.

In any scientific study that purports to show the difference in outcomes as a result of an intervention, it is important that the study group match the control group to the greatest degree possible. In the Smith et al. study, the two groups differed widely. For example, the children in the "untimely" group, as reported by the authors, were from families of lower socioeconomic status than the "timely" group, their families had lower incomes, a smaller percentage of their parents were college graduates, and a higher percentage of their parents were single parents—all factors that correlate with lower neuropsychological testing scores. The authors do acknowledge these factors and claim to have adjusted their findings accordingly, but there is no way to know what adjustment was made and how confounding these differences were to the results. There was also a higher percentage of males in the "untimely" group—58 percent compared to 46.5 percent—another factor associated with lower neuropsychological testing scores. Again, there is no way to know if the authors adequately adjusted for this discrepancy. In the entire study, only nine children were completely unvaccinated and there is no analysis of their outcomes on the testing, so the study actually gives us no information about the difference in neuropsychological health between vaccinated versus unvaccinated children.

Finally, there is no significant information provided in the study as to why the parents decided to delay vaccinating their children. Based on my experience and research, the most frequent reasons parents don't vaccinate their children are that they are too poor or displaced to seek routine medical care (this seems to be the case from the demographic data provided in the study); they have an older child that they think was hurt by vaccines and have therefore decided to delay vaccinating subsequent children; or they are seeing delays or problems in their infants and associate these delays or problems with vaccines and have therefore decided to hold off or delay further vaccines. The

Smith et al. study inadequately explores the reasons behind parental decision making. The problem is that each of these reasons would tend to skew the results toward more children with problems showing up in the "untimely" group. For example, if we are to believe ("if" being an admittedly operative word here) that autism runs in families, then a family with an autistic older sibling is more likely to delay vaccinating younger children if they suspect that vaccines played a role in the autism of the older child. The result of parental decision making, which remains unexplored in the study, is that more vulnerable children will naturally concentrate in the "untimely" group. For these and other reasons—including authorial conflicts of interest—the Smith et al. study doesn't legitimately further our understanding of whether, or to what degree, vaccines contribute to neuropsychological problems in our children.

The other frequently cited study is the "Jain et al. study," often referred to as the "nail in the coffin." This study was published in the *Journal of the American Medical Association* in 2015 under the title "Autism Occurrence by MMR Vaccine Status among US Children with Older Siblings with and without Autism." The study aims to find a connection (or lack of a connection) between the MMR vaccine and autism by age 2, 3, 4, and 5 years old, the presumption being that children who have an older autistic sibling may be more sensitive to the MMR vaccine. As with any study, it is crucial that the cohorts be as similar as possible —in this case, that the results not be confounded because parents are avoiding the MMR vaccine *because* of an older sibling with autism or because they see developing autistic traits in their younger children. This confounding variable is called "healthy user bias" and has been acknowledged by the CDC to be a confounding variable in many studies on vaccines. In fact, the authors of the study acknowledge that this is an important issue in understanding the results of their study: "It is possible, for example, that this pattern is driven by selective parental decision making around MMR immunization, i.e., *parents who notice social or communication delays in their children decide to forestall vaccination* (emphasis added). Because as a group children with recognized delays are likely to be at higher risk of ASD, such selectivity could result in a tendency for some higher-risk children to be unexposed."

The subsequent analysis they provide is complex, but the clearest conclusion one can draw from the data provided is that due to autism-motivated parental behavior (i.e., healthy user bias), autistic children are 38.5 percent less likely to receive the MMR vaccine than nonautistic children. So more MMR-unvaccinated children are autistic *because* their parents avoided the vaccine *because* they were already seeing autistic traits in their children. This is important because when the results are adjusted for this confounding variable, the results in fact show a positive association between the MMR vaccine and autism, not the other way around.

Some claim this study proves that there's no connection between vaccines and autism, but it doesn't even come close to doing so: The children in this study were fully vaccinated with every other vaccine besides MMR. I could go on, dissecting study after study, symposium after symposium, but instead I encourage everyone, particularly those involved in the health care of children either as practitioners or as policy makers, to thoroughly review *Vaccine Papers* (vaccinepapers.org) for the most thorough analysis I've seen to date on vaccine science.

APPENDIX B

Components of Common Vaccines

DTaP (Infanrix)

aluminum hydroxide, bovine extract, formaldehyde or formalin, glutaraldehyde, 2-phenoxyethanol, polysorbate 80

Aluminum. Aluminum is put into vaccines as an adjuvant so that there is a stronger immune (i.e., antibody) reaction. Parenteral (i.e., given by injection) aluminum is known to accumulate in the tissues of the central nervous system and the bones, resulting in significant toxicity.[1] The maximum allowable dose of parenteral aluminum according to the US Food and Drug Administration (FDA) is 25 micrograms (mcg) per day. According to one manufacturer's label, the aluminum content of the following vaccines is:

Hib: 225 mcg
Hepatitis B: 250 mcg
DTaP: 170–625 mcg
Pneumococcus: 125 mcg
Hepatitis A: 250 mcg
HPV: 500 mcg

Pentacel: 1500 mcg
Pediarix: 850 mcg

The amount of aluminum given to newborn babies with their hepatitis B injection is fourteen times the FDA maximum allowable dose for an eight-pound baby. For those following the CDC vaccine schedule at the 2-, 4-, and 6-month checkups, aluminum exceeds 1,000 mcg. Parenteral aluminum has been associated with numerous health issues, including autoimmune diseases,[2] neurological damage,[3] autism,[4] demyelinating disorders such as MS,[5] and others.

Formaledhyde/Formalin. Formaldehyde (or its watery form, called formalin) is commonly used to embalm bodies as they await burial or cremation. It's added to vaccines as a "preservative," supposedly to prevent the deterioration of the active ingredients in the vaccine. The International Agency for Research on Cancer classifies formaldehyde as a human carcinogen[6] and in 2011 the National Toxicology Program named formaldehyde as a known human carcinogen.[7] It is estimated that up to 20 percent of the general population is allergic to formaldehyde and any exposure is enough to trigger allergic symptoms. Furthermore, formaldehyde is oxidized into formic acid, a potent neurotoxin, which can damage both the liver and the kidneys.

Glutaraldehyde. Glutaraldehyde is an organic compound used to disinfect medical and dental equipment. Studies have shown that exposure to glutaraldehyde can be associated with asthma, allergies, respiratory infections, and diarrhea.[8]

2-Phenoxyethanol. 2-Phenoxyethanol is used as an antibiotic in vaccines. According to the material safety data sheet, it is toxic if swallowed and in particular is associated with reproductive abnormalities. The listed side effects include headache, shock, convulsions, weakness, kidney damage, cardiac failure, kidney failure, and death.[9]

Polysorbate 80. Polysorbate 80 is a surfactant, which means it helps substances stay suspended in a solution so they can be evenly distributed. Without polysorbate 80 in vaccines, the components would tend to precipitate out and be harder to inject. It is this same quality in polysorbate 80 that enables substances to cross the blood-brain barrier. This means that every component of the vaccine has greater access to the brain if the vaccine contains polysorbate 80. Research on polysorbate 80 has concluded: "Clinical studies have shown Polysorbate 80 to increase the risk of serious side effects (e.g. blood clots, stroke, heart attack, heart failure) and death in some cases. It has been shown to shorten survival and/or increase the risk of tumor growth or recurrence in patients with certain types of cancer." A study from Slovakia found that injecting rats with polysorbate 80 on days four through seven after birth accelerated their maturation rates, prolonged their estrous cycle, and decreased the adult weight of their uterus and ovaries, all signs of chronic estrogen stimulation. These defects led to an increase in infertility in the injected animals.[10]

DTaP (Tripedia)

aluminum potassium sulfate, ammonium sulfate,
bovine extract, formaldehyde or formalin, gelatin,
polysorbate 80, sodium phosphate

Gelatin. Research by MIT scientist Stephanie Seneff has shown that all commercial gelatin used in the United States is contaminated with the herbicide glyphosate (Roundup) as a result of current animal-feeding practices. Dr. Zach Bush has shown that glyphosate increases the zonulin production in the gut lumen, increasing permeability of the gut wall, a crucial step in the pathogenesis of autoimmune diseases. The gelatin in vaccines is used to grow the microorganisms that are contained in the vaccine.

DTaP-IPV (Kinrix)

aluminum hydroxide, bovine extract, formaldehyde,
lactalbumin hydrolysate, monkey kidney tissue,
neomycin sulfate, polymyxin B, polysorbate 80

Lactalbumin hydrolysate. Lactalbumin, which is also used as a medium for growing microorganisms, is a foreign protein that our digestive system is designed to keep out of our blood. When foreign proteins enter the bloodstream, the body reacts by producing antibodies. It is these antibodies produced in response to the introduction of foreign proteins in our bloodstream that provoke autoimmune diseases. Lactalbumin is one such foreign protein in vaccines capable of inducing autoimmune reactions.

Monkey kidney tissue. This is another medium used to grow the organisms contained in the vaccine, and it is thought to be a source of the virus SV-40, an oncogenic (cancer-causing) virus. The injection of monkey kidney tissue is suspected to be a possible source of the increase of childhood cancers, especially leukemia.

Neomycin sulfate and polymyxin B. These are two common antibiotics used to help sterilize a vaccine. At this time there has not been significant research into the routine injection of antibiotics into young children. All antibiotics interfere with the development of a healthy microbiome (see chapter 4).

DTaP-Hep B-IPV (Pediarix)

aluminum hydroxide, aluminum phosphate,
bovine protein, lactalbumin hydrolysate, formaldehyde
or formalin, glutaraldehyde, monkey kidney tissue,
neomycin, 2-phenoxyethanol, polymycin B,
polysorbate 80, yeast protein

Yeast protein. Yeast protein is the name used for various forms of processed yeast. All yeast extracts contain monosodium L-glutamate (MSG), a known neurotoxin. The symptoms associated with MSG include headaches, sleep issues, irritable bowel syndrome, asthma, diabetes, dementia, attention-deficit/hyperactivity disorder, seizures, stroke, and allergic reactions. Most vaccines contain some amount of MSG because they are grown on nutrient bases, which contain up to 10 percent glutamic acid, the precursor of MSG.

Hib/Hep B (Comvax)

amino acids, aluminum hydroxyphosphate, sulfate, dextrose, formaldehyde or formalin, mineral salts, sodium borate, soy peptone, yeast protein

Soy peptone. Soy peptone is a soy protein medium that a virus in a vaccine can be grown on. Many people today are allergic to soy and soy products. It's possible that the parenteral injections of soy proteins within vaccines received as children are partially responsible for sensitizing people to react against proteins from soy.

HPV (Cervarix)

3-O-desacyl-4'-monophosphoryl lipid A (MPL), aluminum hydroxide, amino acids, insect cell protein, mineral salts, sodium dihydrogen phosphate dihydrate, vitamins

3-O-desacyl-4'-monophosphoryl lipid A and insect cell protein. There is not much information about these two new components except that they are proprietary adjuvants used by GlaxoSmithKline in the preparation of its vaccines. Like all adjuvants used to stimulate an immune response, they are pieces of protein or lipids from animals or plants that cause an immunological reaction when injected into humans.

HPV (Gardasil)

amino acids, amorphous aluminum hydroxyphosphate sulfate, carbohydrates, L-histidine, mineral salts, polysorbate 80, sodium borate, vitamins

L-histidine. Histidine is considered an essential amino acid, but its toxicity when administered parenterally within a vaccine is unknown. The FDA states that due to this uncertainty L-histidine is not to be given to pregnant or nursing mothers.

Influenza (Fluvirin)

beta-propiolactone, egg protein, neomycin, polymyxin B, polyloxyethylene 9-10 nonyl phenol (triton N-101, octoxynol 9), thimerosal

Egg protein. Eggs are one of the most allergenic foods. Incidence of egg allergies has increased in the vaccine era. Injecting egg proteins in children at an early age is one method of sensitizing them against this protein for life, in essence provoking an allergic reaction to eggs.

Thimerosal. Thimerosal is the preservative form of mercury. It is added to vaccines primarily to prevent bacterial growth, as most forms of mercury have potent antibiotic effects. While thimerosal was technically removed from most (not all) vaccines in 2004, thimerosal is still used in the vaccine creation process and then is "filtered out" with only "trace" amounts remaining. For perspective:[11]

2 parts per billion (ppb) mercury is the mandated limit in drinking water.

200 ppb mercury in liquid waste renders it a toxic hazard.
2,000 ppb mercury in flu vaccines is considered a "trace" amount.
50,000 ppb mercury in multidose flu vaccines is given to infants, pregnant women, and everyone else.

Mercury is a known and potent neurotoxin, one that, when given access to the central nervous system, causes neuronal deterioration, confirmed by decades of research. Furthermore, mercury exposure has been directly linked to autism in the developing child. A 2003 study published in the journal *Pediatric Rehabilitation* states: "This study provides additional epidemiological evidence for a link between increasing mercury from thimerosal-containing childhood vaccines and neurodevelopmental disorders."[12] For a review of the many studies linking mercury/thimerosal exposure with neurodevelopmental issues in children, I recommend *Miller's Review of Critical Vaccine Studies*.

MMR (MMR-II)

amino acid, bovine albumin or serum, chick embryo fibroblasts, human serum albumin, gelatin, monosodium L-glutamate, neomycin, phosphate buffers, sorbitol, sucrose, vitamins

The MMR vaccine contains three live viruses, all of which need to be grown on biological media. In the case of this particular vaccine, the media come from free amino acids and proteins from cows, chickens, and aborted fetuses. Injecting proteins or their amino acid components is one way to provoke antibody-mediated autoimmune reactions.

MMRV (ProQuad)

bovine albumin or serum, gelatin, human serum albumin, monosodium L-glutamate, MRC-5 cellular protein, neomycin,

sodium phosphate dibasic, sodium bicarbonate,
sorbitol, sucrose, potassium phosphate monobasic,
potassium chloride, potassium

MRC-5. MRC-5 is derived from tissue obtained from aborted
human fetuses. One factor that can perpetuate the autoimmune process is spillage of DNA from inside the cell into the
blood when organ tissue is destroyed. This free DNA needs
to be targeted and eliminated by the same immune response
leading to a cycle of tissue destruction, leakage of DNA, and
then more antibodies to eliminate the free DNA, which then
leads to more destruction of tissue. A study by Dr. Helen
Ratajczak found that autism rates soared in 1995 following
the introduction of nontyped human DNA into vaccines.[13]
With blood transfusions, the recipient must be "typed" for
compatibility with the donor; this "typing" is not done with
vaccines, even though using MRC-5 in vaccination is a form
of introducing human DNA into another person.

Monosodium L-glutamate (MSG). Most people are familiar
with "Chinese restaurant syndrome," a result of exposure to
the MSG used in some Chinese restaurants. Many people
are extremely sensitive to even minute amounts of MSG,
even when it is orally ingested. Giving MSG by injection is
worse. The common symptoms of MSG exposure include
headaches, seizures, asthma, and neurodevelopmental delays
that can arise with long-term exposure.

Rotavirus (RotaTeq)

cell culture media, fetal bovine serum, sodium citrate,
sodium diphosphate monobasic monohydrate,
sodium hydroxide sucrose, polysorbate 80

This vaccine is given to combat a common cause of diarrhea in
infants and young children.

Tdap (Boostrix)

aluminum phosphate, formaldehyde or formalin,
glutaraldehyde, 2-phenoxyethanol

This is the basic booster shot given to children in four additional
doses according to the CDC schedule.

Varicella (Varivax)

bovine albumin or serum, ethylenediamine-tetraacetic acid
sodium (EDTA), gelatin, monosodium L-glutamate,
MRC-5 DNA and cellular protein, neomycin, potassium
chloride, potassium phosphate monobasic, sodium
phosphate monobasic, sucrose

This is the standard chicken pox vaccine, the components of
which have been discussed previously.

RECOMMENDED RESOURCES

Books

Campbell-McBride, Natasha. *Gut and Psychology Syndrome: Natural Treatment for Autism, Dyspraxia, A.D.D., Dyslexia, A.D.H.D., Depression, Schizophrenia.* 2nd Edition. White River Junction, VT: Chelsea Green Publishing, 2010.

Cowan, Thomas S., Sally Fallon Morell, and Jaimen McMillan. *The Fourfold Path to Healing.* Washington, DC: NewTrends Publishing, 2004.

Elsegood, Linda, ed. *The LDN Book: How a Little-Known Generic Drug—Low Dose Naltrexone—Could Revolutionize Treatment for Autoimmune Diseases, Cancer, Autism, Depression, and More.* White River Junction, VT: Chelsea Green Publishing, 2016.

Ho, Mae-Wan. *The Rainbow and the Worm: The Physics of Organisms.* Singapore: World Scientific Publishing Company, 2008.

Humphries, Suzanne, and Roman Bystrianyk. *Dissolving Illusions: Disease, Vaccines, and the Forgotten History.* CreateSpace Independent Publishing Platform, 2013.

Illich, Ivan. *Deschooling Society.* New York City: Harper Perennial, 1972.

———. *Medical Nemesis.* New York City: Pantheon Books, 1972.

Katz, Sandor Ellix. *The Art of Fermentation: An In-Depth Exploration of Essential Concepts and Processes from around the World*. White River Junction, VT: Chelsea Green Publishing, 2012.

———. *Wild Fermentation: The Flavor, Nutrition, and Craft of Live-Culture Foods*. 2nd Edition. White River Junction, VT: Chelsea Green Publishing, 2016.

Leons-Weiler, James. *The Environmental and Genetic Causes of Autism*. New York City: Skyhorse Publishing, 2016.

Ling, Gilbert N. *Life at the Cell and Below-Cell Level: The Hidden History of a Fundamental Revolution in Biology*. Nampa, ID: Pacific Press, 2001.

Miller, Neil. *Miller's Review of Critical Vaccine Studies: 400 Important Scientific Papers Summarized for Parents and Researchers*. Santa Fe, NM: New Atlantean Press, 2016.

Morell, Sally Fallon, and Thomas S. Cowan. *The Nourishing Traditions Book of Baby and Child Care*. Washington, DC: New Trends Publishing, 2013.

Morell, Sally Fallon, and Mary G. Enig. *Nourishing Traditions: The Cookbook That Challenges Politically Correct Nutrition and Diet Dictocrats*. 2nd Revised Edition. Washington, DC: NewTrends Publishing, n.d.

Pollack, Gerald H. *Cells, Gels and the Engines of Life: A New Unifying Approach to Cell Function*. Seattle: Ebner and Sons Publishing, 2001.

———. *The Fourth Phase of Water: Beyond Solid, Liquid, Vapor*. Seattle: Ebner and Sons Publishing, 2013.

Documentaries

Pilaro, Chris, and Kendall Nelson. *The Greater Good*. BNP Pictures, 2011.

Wakefield, Andrew. *Vaxxed: From Cover-up to Catastrophe*. Burbank, CA: Cinema Libre Studio, 2016.

Products

Low Dose Naltrexone

The best approach to obtaining a prescription for low dose naltrexone is to consult the website www.lowdosenaltrexone.org. There you will find a list of pharmacies that compound it and practitioners who prescribe it. You can also purchase good-quality 4.5-milligram capsules of naltrexone from www.antiaging-systems.com.

Colostrum

There are many good sources for powdered colostrum. I generally use www.rawrevelations.com.

Restore Soil-Derived Mineral Supplement
www.shop.restore4life.com

Andreas Seed Oils
www.andreasseedoils.com

Adya Clarity Water Purification and Filtration System
www.adyawater.com

Tribest Duet Water Revitalizer
www.tribestlife.com

Miron Glass
www.miron-glas.com

Flaska Water Bottles
www.flaska.us

Weston A. Price Foundation Shopping Guide
www.westonaprice.org/about-us/shopping-guide/

NOTES

Introduction

1. "Vaccine Requirements vs. Federal Vaccine Recommendations," National Vaccine Information Center, 2018.
2. "Technavio Expects the Global Human Vaccines Market to Reach Close to USD 61 Billion by 2020," Business Wire, 2016.

Chapter 1: The Changing Nature of Childhood Illness

1. Michelle Perro and Vincanne Adams, *What's Making Our Children Sick?: How Industrial Food Is Causing an Epidemic of Chronic Illness, and What Parents (and Doctors) Can Do About It* (White River Junction, VT: Chelsea Green Publishing, 2017), 7.
2. "Autism Spectrum Disorder (ASD)," Data & Statistics, Centers for Disease Control and Prevention, 2012.
3. Perro and Adams, *What's Making Our Children Sick?*
4. "Most Recent Asthma Data," Centers for Disease Control and Prevention, 2017.
5. Perro and Adams, *What's Making Our Children Sick?*, ix.
6. Benjamin Zablotsky, Lindsey I. Black, and Stephen J. Blumberg, "Estimated Prevalence of Children with Diagnosed Developmental Disabilities in the United States, 2014–2016," National Center for Health Statistics, 2017.

Chapter 2: Fever and the Nature of Acute Disease

1. Edward F. McCarthy, "The Toxins of William B. Coley and the Treatment of Bone and Soft-Tissue Sarcomas," *Iowa Orthopaedic Journal* 26 (2006): 154–58.

2. Carl Engelking, "Germ of an Idea: William Coley's Cancer-Killing Toxins," *Discover Magazine*, 2016.

3. McCarthy, "The Toxins of William B. Coley."

4. These figures come from personal communication with Helen Coley Nauts, founder of the Cancer Research Institute and daughter of William B. Coley.

5. Engelking, "Germ of an Idea."

6. Ibid.

7. McCarthy, "The Toxins of William B. Coley."

8. Ibid.

9. Ibid; and Ed Yong, "The Most Promising Cancer Therapy in Decades Is About to Get Better," *Atlantic*, 2016.

Chapter 3: Our Immune System(s)

1. Peter Good, "Did Acetaminophen Provoke the Autism Epidemic?" *Alternative Medicine Review: A Journal of Clinical Therapeutic* 14, no. 4 (2009): 364–72; and Stephen T. Schultz, et al., "Acetaminophen (Paracetamol) Use, Measles-Mumps-Rubella Vaccination, and Autistic Disorder: The Results of a Parent Survey," *Autism: The International Journal of Research and Practice* 12, no. 3 (2008): 293–307.

2. W. H. Havinga, "Managing Measles. Giving Paracetamol for Fever Is Unnecessary," *BMJ: British Medical Journal* 314, no. 7095 (1997): 1692–93; and M. A. Phadke, P. V. Paranjape, and A. S. Joshi, "Ibuprofen in Children with Infective Disorders—Antipyretic Efficacy," *British Journal of Clinical Practice* 39, no. 11–12 (1985): 437–40.

3. Ken Tsumiyama, Yumi Miyazaki, and Shunichi Shiozawa, "Self-Organized Criticality Theory of Autoimmunity," *PLoS ONE* 4, no. 12 (2009).

4. Carlo Perricone, et al., "Autoimmune/Inflammatory Syndrome Induced by Adjuvants (ASIA) 2013: Unveiling the Pathogenic, Clinical and Diagnostic Aspects," *Journal of Autoimmunity* 47 (2013): 1–16; and Alessandra

Soriano, Gideon Nesher, and Yehuda Shoenfeld,
"Predicting Post-Vaccination Autoimmunity: Who
Might Be at Risk?" *Pharmacological Research* 92 (2015):
18–22.

Chapter 4: Autoimmunity and the Gut

1. Tim Spector, "What a Hunter-Gatherer Diet Does to the
Body," CNN, 2017.
2. Ibid.
3. Raymond MacDougall, "NIH Human Microbiome Project
Defines Normal Bacterial Makeup of the Body," National
Institutes of Health, 2012.
4. Ron Sender, Shai Fuchs, and Ron Milo, "Are We Really
Vastly Outnumbered? Revisiting the Ratio of Bacterial to
Host Cells in Humans," *Cell* 164, no. 3 (2016): 337–40.
5. Mei Chien Chua, et al., "Effect of Synbiotic on the Gut
Microbiota of Cesarean Delivered Infants: A
Randomized, Double-Blind, Multicenter Study," *Journal
of Pediatric Gastroenterology and Nutrition* 65, no. 1
(2017): 102.
6. Stephanie Seneff, "Why We Need to Reexamine the Risk/
Benefit Tradeoffs of Vaccines," *Wise Traditions in Food,
Farming and the Healing Arts*, (Summer 2015).
7. Alessio Fasano, "Zonulin and Its Regulation of Intestinal
Barrier Function: The Biological Door to Inflammation,
Autoimmunity, and Cancer," *Physiological Reviews* 91, no. 1
(2011): 151–75.
8. Kate O'Rourke, "Study Hints Gut Microbiome Plays a Role
in Multiple Sclerosis," *Gastroenterology & Endoscopy News*,
2014.
9. Bret Stetka, "Could Multiple Sclerosis Begin in the Gut?"
Scientific American, 2014; and Pavan Bhargava and Ellen
M. Mowry, "Gut Microbiome and Multiple Sclerosis,"
Current Neurology and Neuroscience Reports 14, no. 10
(2014): 492.

Chapter 6: Rethinking Cell Biology

1. Gerald H. Pollack, *The Fourth Phase of Water: Beyond Solid, Liquid, Vapor* (Seattle, WA: Ebner and Sons Publishing, 2013).

Chapter 8: The Chicken Pox Vaccine

1. Sandra S. Chaves, et al., "Loss of Vaccine-Induced Immunity to Varicella over Time," *New England Journal of Medicine* 356, no. 11 (2007): 1121–29.
2. "Monitoring the Impact of Varicella Vaccination," Centers for Disease Control and Prevention, 2016.
3. Erkki Pesonen, et al., "Dual Role of Infections as Risk Factors for Coronary Heart Disease," *Atherosclerosis* 192, no. 2 (2007): 370–75.
4. Graciela Gutierrez, "History of Chicken Pox May Reduce Risk of Brain Cancer Later in Life," Baylor College of Medicine, 2016.
5. "Shingles Surveillance," Centers for Disease Control and Prevention, 2017.
6. W. Katherine Yih, et al., "The Incidence of Varicella and Herpes Zoster in Massachusetts as Measured by the Behavioral Risk Factor Surveillance System (BRFSS) during a Period of Increasing Varicella Vaccine Coverage, 1998–2003," *BMC Public Health* 5 (2005): 68.
7. M. Brisson, et al., "Exposure to Varicella Boosts Immunity to Herpes-Zoster: Implications for Mass Vaccination against Chickenpox," *Vaccine* 20, no. 19–20 (2002): 2500–2507.
8. Yih, et al., "The Incidence of Varicella and Herpes Zoster in Massachusetts."
9. G. S. Goldman, "Cost-Benefit Analysis of Universal Varicella Vaccination in the U.S. Taking into Account the Closely Related Herpes-Zoster Epidemiology," *Vaccine* 23, no. 25 (2005): 3349–55.
10. Sara L. Thomas, Jeremy G. Wheeler, and Andrew J. Hall, "Contacts with Varicella or with Children and Protection

against Herpes Zoster in Adults: A Case-Control Study,"
Lancet 360, no. 9334 (2002): 678–82.

11. Colleen Chun, et al., "Laboratory Characteristics of
Suspected Herpes Zoster in Vaccinated Children," *Pediatric
Infectious Disease Journal* 30, no. 8 (2011): 719–21.

12. Ibid.

13. G. S. Goldman and P. G. King, "Review of the United
States Universal Varicella Vaccination Program: Herpes
Zoster Incidence Rates, Cost-Effectiveness, and Vaccine
Efficacy Based Primarily on the Antelope Valley Varicella
Active Surveillance Project Data," *Vaccine* 31, no. 13
(2013): 1680–94.

14. Eric Sagonowsky, "Merck's Zostavax Draws New Litigation
from Patients Alleging They Contracted Shingles,"
FiercePharma, 2017.

15. Wellington Sun and US Food and Drug Administration,
Letter to Merck Sharp & Dohme Corp., "August 28, 2014
Approval Letter—ZOSTAVAX," 2014.

16. Sagonowsky, "Merck's Zostavax Draws New Litigation."

17. R. E. Fried, "Herpes Zoster," *New England Journal of
Medicine*, no. 18 (2013): 369.

18. Yi Chun Lai and Yik Weng Yew, "Severe Autoimmune
Adverse Events Post Herpes Zoster Vaccine: A Case-
Control Study of Adverse Events in a National Database,"
Journal of Drugs in Dermatology 14, no. 7 (2015): 681–84.

19. Eric Sagonowsky, "Zostavax Patients Sue Merck, Claiming
Shingles Shot Caused Injuries and Death," FiercePharma,
2017.

20. Sagonowsky, "Merck's Zostavax Draws New Litigation."

21. Eric Sagonowsky, "GlaxoSmithKline's Bexsero, Shingrix to
Pass $1B Sales Mark by 2022: Report," FiercePharma, 2017.

22. J.B. Handley, "10 Reasons CDC Employees Should Be
'Crying in the Hallways,'" *Medium* (blog), 2017.

23. Ibid.

24. Ibid.

Chapter 9: The Polio Vaccine

1. "What Is Polio?" Centers for Disease Control and Prevention, 2017.

2. Dan Olmsted, "The Age of Polio Series: Explosion," *Age of Autism: Daily Web Newspaper of Autism Epidemic* (blog), 2016; and Dan Olmsted and Mark Blaxill, "The Age of Polio: How an Old Virus and New Toxins Triggered a Man-Made Epidemic," *Age of Autism: Daily Web Newspaper of Autism Epidemic* (blog), 2011.

3. Ibid.

4. Ibid.

5. Ibid.

6. Ibid.

7. Ibid.

8. Douglas M. Considine, *Van Nostrand's Scientific Encyclopedia*, Fifth Edition, 1775, (Ann Arbor, MI: Van Nostrand Reinhold, 1995).

9. Olmsted, "The Age of Polio Series: Explosion"; and Olmsted and Blaxill, "The Age of Polio."

10. Marco Cáceres, "How Scientific Was the Identification of the Poliovirus?" *The Vaccine Reaction* (blog), 2017.

11. "What Is Polio?" Centers for Disease Control and Prevention, 2017.

12. Søren Wengel Mogensen, et al., "The Introduction of Diphtheria-Tetanus-Pertussis and Oral Polio Vaccine among Young Infants in an Urban African Community: A Natural Experiment," *EBioMedicine* 17 (2017): 192–98.

13. Morton S. Biskind, "Public Health Aspects of the New Insecticides," *American Journal of Digestive Diseases* 20, no. 11 (1953): 331–41.

14. Olmsted, "The Age of Polio Series: Explosion"; and Olmsted and Blaxill, "The Age of Polio."

15. Daniel Dresden, *Physiological Investigations into the Action of DDT* (Arnhem, Netherlands: G. W. Van Der Wiel & Co., 1949).

16. Ralph R. Scobey, "The Poison Cause of Poliomyelitis and Obstructions to Its Investigation," *Archives of Pediatrics* 69, no. 4 (1952): 172–93.

17. Biskind, "Public Health Aspects of the New Insecticides."

18. Public Law 518, *Federal Statutes*, Volume 68, 1954, p. 511. Public Law 905, *Federal Statutes*, 1956.

19. G. C. Brown, W. R. Lenz, and G. H. Agate, "Laboratory Data on the Detroit Poliomyelitis Epidemic—1958," *Journal of the American Medical Association* 172 (1960): 807–12.

Chapter 10: The Measles Vaccine

1. Yasuhiko Kubota, et al., "Association of Measles and Mumps with Cardiovascular Disease: The Japan Collaborative Cohort (JACC) Study," *Atherosclerosis* 241, no. 2 (2015): 682–86; M. L. Newhouse, et al., "A Case Control Study of Carcinoma of the Ovary," *British Journal of Preventive & Social Medicine* 31, no. 3 (1977): 148–53; K. F. Kölmel, O. Gefeller, and B. Haferkamp, "Febrile Infections and Malignant Melanoma: Results of a Case-Control Study," *Melanoma Research* 2, no. 3 (1992): 207–11; H. U. Albonico, H. U. Bräker, and J. Hüsler, "Febrile Infectious Childhood Diseases in the History of Cancer Patients and Matched Controls," *Medical Hypotheses* 51, no. 4 (1998): 315–20; and Maurizio Montella, et al., "Do Childhood Diseases Affect NHL and HL Risk? A Case-Control Study from Northern and Southern Italy," *Leukemia Research* 30, no. 8 (2006): 917–22.

2. "The Story of . . . Smallpox—and Other Deadly Eurasian Germs," PBS.org, 2005.

3. Physicians for Informed Consent, "Disease Information Statement, Measles: What Parents Need to Know," updated December 2017.

4. T. C. Merigan and D. A. Stevens. "Viral Infections in Man Associated with Acquired Immunological Deficiency States," *Federation Proceedings* 30, no. 6 (1971): 1858–64.

Chapter 11: Basic Autoimmune Treatment Protocol for Children and Adults

1. Søren Wengel Mogensen, et al., "The Introduction of Diphtheria-Tetanus-Pertussis and Oral Polio Vaccine among Young Infants in an Urban African Community: A Natural Experiment," *EBioMedicine* 17 (2017): 192–98. doi:10.1016/j.ebiom.2017.01.041.
2. Alessio Fasano, "Zonulin, Regulation of Tight Junctions, and Autoimmune Diseases," *Annals of the New York Academy of Sciences* 1258, no. 1 (2012): 25–33.
3. Sydney Spiesel, Dara Kass, and Brian Thomas Fletcher, "Tales from the Nursery," *Slate*, 2006.

Conclusion

1. Sally Fallon Morell and Thomas S. Cowan, *The Nourishing Traditions Book of Baby & Child Care* (Washington, DC: NewTrends Publishing, 2013).
2. Institute of Medicine Vaccine Safety Committee, "Death," in *Adverse Events Associated with Childhood Vaccines: Evidence Bearing on Causality*, edited by Kathleen R. Stratton, Cynthia J. Howe, and Richard B. Johnston (Washington, DC: National Academies Press, 1994).

Appendix A

1. Micahel J. Smith and Charles R. Woods, "On-time Vaccine Receipt in the First Year Does Not Adversely Affect Neuropsychological Outcomes," *Pediatrics* 125, no. 6 (2010).

Appendix B

1. Department of Health and Human Services, Food and Drug Administration, Document NDA 12-626/S-019, Federal Food, Drug and Cosmetic Act for Dextrose Injections.
2. "Hyperstimulation of the immune system by various (vaccine) adjuvants, including aluminum, carries an inherent risk for serious autoimmune disorders affecting

the central nervous system." Christopher A. Shaw and L. Tomljenovic, "Aluminum in the Central Nervous System (CNS): Toxicity in Humans and Animals, Vaccine Adjuvants, and Autoimmunity," *Immunologic Research* 56, no. 2–3 (2013): 304–16.

3. Ibid.

4. "Our results . . . suggest that a causal relationship may exist between the amount of [aluminum] administered to preschool children at various ages through vaccination and the rising prevalence of [autism spectrum disorders]." Lucija Tomljenovic and Christopher A. Shaw, "Do Aluminum Vaccine Adjuvants Contribute to the Rising Prevalence of Autism?" *Journal of Inorganic Biochemistry* 105, no. 11 (2011): 1489–99.

5. "On the grounds of our clinical and experimental data, we believe that increased attention should be paid to possible long-term neurologic effects of continuously escalating doses of alum-containing vaccines administered to the general population." R. K. Gherardi and F. J. Authier, "Macrophagic Myofasciitis: Characterization and Pathophysiology," *Lupus* 21, no. 2 (2012): 184–89.

6. International Agency for Research on Cancer Working Group on the Evaluation of Carcinogenic Risks to Humans, "Formaldehyde, 2-Butoxyethanol and 1-Tert-Butoxypropan-2-Ol," *IARC Monographs on the Evaluation of Carcinogenic Risks to Humans* 88 (2006): 1–478.

7. National Toxicology Program, "NTP 12th Report on Carcinogens," *Report on Carcinogens: Carcinogen Profiles* 12 (2011): iii–499.

8. Scott M. Ravis, et al., "Glutaraldehyde-Induced and Formaldehyde-Induced Allergic Contact Dermatitis among Dental Hygienists and Assistants," *Journal of the American Dental Association* 134, no. 8 (2003): 1072–78; S. Quirce, et al., "Glutaraldehyde-Induced Asthma," *Allergy* 54, no. 10 (1999): 1121–22; Errol Zeiger, Bhaskar Gollapudi, and

Pamela Spencer, "Genetic Toxicity and Carcinogenicity
Studies of Glutaraldehyde—A Review," *Mutation Research*
589, no. 2 (2005): 136–51; and Shahla Azadi, Kimberly J.
Klink, and B. Jean Meade, "Divergent Immunological
Responses Following Glutaraldehyde Exposure," *Toxicology
and Applied Pharmacology* 197, no. 1 (2004): 1–8.

9. "2-Phenoxyethanol MSDS," Material Safety Data Sheet,
ScienceLab.com, 2013.

10. "Polysorbate 80 Risks," *Vaccine Choice Canada* (blog),
2013.

11. "Mercury in Vaccines FAQs," National Vaccine Information
Center, 2018.

12. David A. Geier and Mark R. Geier, "An Assessment of the
Impact of Thimerosal on Childhood Neurodevelopmental
Disorders," *Pediatric Rehabilitation* 6, no. 2 (2003):
97–102.

13. Helen V. Ratajczak, "Theoretical Aspects of Autism:
Causes—A Review," *Journal of Immunotoxicology* 8, no. 1
(2011): 68–79.

INDEX

Note: Page numbers in *italics* refer to charts.

ABOUT THE AUTHOR

Thomas Cowan, MD, has studied and written about many subjects in medicine, including nutrition, homeopathy, anthroposophical medicine, and herbal medicine. He is the author of *Human Heart, Cosmic Heart*, principal author of *The Fourfold Path to Healing*, and co-author (with Sally Fallon Morell) of *The Nourishing Traditions Book of Baby and Child Care*. Dr. Cowan has served as vice president of the Physicians' Association for Anthroposophic Medicine and is a founding board member of the Weston A. Price Foundation. He also writes the "Ask the Doctor" column in *Wise Traditions in Food, Farming, and the Healing Arts* (the Weston A. Price Foundation's quarterly magazine), has lectured throughout the United States and Canada, and is the co-founder of a family business, Dr. Cowan's Garden. He has three grown children and currently practices medicine in San Francisco, where he resides with his wife, Lynda Smith.

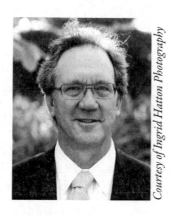

Courtesy of Ingrid Hatton Photography

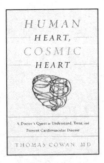
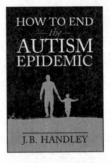
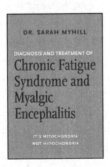
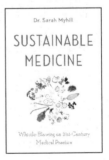
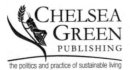